Recovering at Home
with a Heart Condition

The Howard A. Rusk Institute
of Rehabilitation Medicine

Recovering at Home with a Heart Condition

A Practical Guide for You
and Your Family

By Florence Weiner,
Mathew H. M. Lee, M.D., F.A.C.P.,
and Harriet Bell, Ph.D.

THE BODY PRESS / PERIGEE

The Client Bill of Rights is used by permission from the Foundation for Hospice and Homecare.

This book provides practical solutions for people recovering at home with a heart condition and their families and caregivers. The authors believe strongly in the vital role of the individual in his/her recovery. However, this book does not attempt to replace your physician. Responsibility for any adverse effects or unforeseen consequences from the use of the information contained in this book is expressly disclaimed by the publisher and the authors.

The Body Press/Perigee Books
are published by
The Berkley Publishing Group
200 Madison Avenue
New York, NY 10016

Library of Congress Cataloging-in-Publication Data

Weiner, Florence.
    Recovering at home with a heart condition : a
practical guide for you and your family / by Florence
Weiner, Mathew H.M. Lee, and Harriet Bell.
        p.   cm.
    Includes bibliographical references and index.
    ISBN 0-399-51844-4
    1. Heart—Diseases—Patients—Rehabilitation. 2. Heart—
Diseases—Patients—Home care. I. Lee,   Mathew H. M.,
date. II. Bell, Harriet. III. Title.
    362.1'9612—dc20   93-32926 CIP

Cover design by Judith Kazdym Leeds

Printed in the United States of America
1   2   3   4   5   6   7   8   9   10

Acknowledgments

The professional excellence and encouragement of the rehabilitation medical staff, physical therapists, occupational therapists, and psychologists of the Rusk Institute made this book possible.

The insights and recommendations of our professional and consumer advisers made the material more useful.

The wisdom and firsthand experiences of men and women with heart conditions ultimately shaped this book.

We are indebted to each of them.

Contents

Chapter Six **Getting Back to Work**   131

Chapter Seven **Being Safe**   145

Chapter Eight **Travel**   163

Chapter Nine **Information, Services, and Products**   171

Foreword

When Dr. Howard A. Rusk pioneered the concept of rehabilitation medicine, he recognized and appreciated the miraculous potential strengths of the human body. The mending, recuperating, and restoration that take place after you leave the hospital is possible because of these strengths.

During the past few years, many popular and professional books, articles, and research studies have examined the mind–body relationship. Dr. Rusk's contribution to rehabilitation medicine was amazing in its concept, nearly fifty years ago, of the unified strength of the body with the mind. This power enables a person to do even better at home than if the individual had remained in the hospital.

The heart is the most studied organ of the body. Even before Hippocrates, the one internal organ that primitive man could feel in himself, see in animals, and identify with, was the heart.

The organ perceived as vital to life was the heart. Since prehistoric times, the heart has been considered as much more than an extraordinarily powerful pump. The heart has been considered the source of emotions, sensitivity, courage, love, loyalty, and compassion.

A person's intellect, imagination, sincerity, romantic inclinations, and affection are linked, in every language and culture, with the heart.

Everyone's vocabulary is filled with heart expressions.

To hearten is to encourage. To do a person's heart good is to make the person happy. To speak from the bottom of your heart is the ultimate in sincerity and appreciation. To have your heart in the right place is to be well-intentioned. There are dozens of other examples; you probably have your own favorite "heartfelt" expression.

Many of these expressions, including those in ancient poems and plays, are in tune with contemporary medicine. They link the heart with the mind, as well as with the entire body.

Dr. Rusk, who is often called the "father of rehabilitation medicine," emphasized that maximum restoration of functions of individuals encompasses not only their physical, but also their social, psychological, and vocational needs.

Rehabilitation medicine was called the third phase of medicine, after primary prevention and diagnosis and treatment.

Much of the initial care for major medical conditions is usually provided in a hospital setting. The trend in medical practice today is toward early discharge and home care therapy. Recuperation takes place at home. Newer technologies and economic considerations have made this both possible and increasingly essential.

Current medical philosophy is to get a patient with almost any medical condition—from childbirth to fractures to cardiac surgery—out of bed as early as possible. A major reason is that a normally functioning heart, as compared to a quiescent heart, is more likely to help the entire body in its recovery. So getting up and out of bed is particularly important for a person with a heart condition.

When you were in the hospital, your doctor and others spoke with you and gave you materials about exercise, nutrition, medication, and other basics for your recovery. Even if they tried to personalize this material, chances are it includes many generalizations. In fact, even those doctors who know you well cannot predict the infinite number of changes and adaptations that will be required because of your personal living situation.

For example, no one can predict how helpful or stressful the members of your family will be, ranging from supportive spouses to members of the family with their own needs, such as teenage or adult children.

Perhaps your physician will tell you to take it easy during the first few weeks at home. Some family members may misinterpret this advice and coddle you.

At the other extreme, whatever information you have already received is likely to be oriented to pushing you to do more than you otherwise might. For every person, there is always that hard-to-find line between necessary exertion and excessive effort.

Dr. Rusk was one of the first physicians to recruit in one place a team of physicians and other rehabilitation specialists. I will always remember the sound of Dr. Rusk's voice as he reiterated, "The most important person on the team is none of us. It is the patient!"

As you read this book—and any other book or article about cardiac rehabilitation—you will be able to decide what is appropriate for you at this particular time. You will find the proper mix of advice and techniques will vary as you go on in your recovery. So, to use a relevant metaphor, "Let your heart be the guide."

About 3 million Americans currently are over the age of eighty-five. An amazingly large number of these men and women do not live in nursing homes or other institutions. They either live alone in their own homes or in the homes of their children or other relatives.

Many of these people drive cars, go shopping, and have active lives. It's a reminder of the remarkable strength of the human body and mind, a tribute to the wonders of modern medicine. So, assuming that you are considerably younger than these men and women aged eighty-five and up, keep them in mind as an inspiring goal.

If that's too much of a reach, find someone else to set up as a model. The ideal prototype is a person your age and with similar circumstances who returned from the hospital a short time ago and now is back at work. You'll find information about support groups throughout this book, and many of the members fit this description.

For many years, Dr. Rusk wrote an unusual column (which appeared in *The New York Times* and other newspapers)—solely about rehabilitation medicine. He once told me that the most common questions from readers involved how to get started when moving from the hospital to the home.

In the thirty-five years I have been practicing medicine, I have been asked the same questions—whether the person is rich or poor, educated or uneducated, the concern is always, "When will I be able to be independent again? What do I have to do to get back to being myself?"

The responsibility of the medical team is not merely to save lives and help you live longer, but to improve your quality of life. That's the essence of rehabilitation medicine. To treat the whole person, one must treat the intertwined physical, emotional, and spiritual needs. Thousands of rehabilitation therapists throughout the world have been trained at the Rusk Institute or have been influenced by this philosophy of the whole person and independent living.

It was only a few decades ago that the concept of rehabilitation medicine meant that you had to remain within a rehabilitation facility for a very long period of time in order to have access to the facility's professionals, resources, and equipment. Today, the resources of rehabilitation institutions are an essential part of the treatment of many medical conditions, particularly for spinal cord and orthopedic injuries, neuromuscular diseases, cardiovascular conditions, and strokes. However, the new orientation is to help a person to get well enough to leave a hospital or rehabilitation facility as soon as possible.

This book, then, is a distillation of fifty years of work with many thousands of people within a hospital environment, with an orientation that focuses not on the hospital but on the home.

This book is for your use at home. That's why we never use the word "patient." We also try to avoid professional jargon. Though you may already know many medical terms, and while you should understand everything that your doctor says to you, you won't find terms such as M.I. (for myocardial infarction, or heart attack) in this book. The reason: We want to provide a book that is as accessible, understandable, and useful as possible. We want to be as supportive and empowering as you will allow us.

We also are concerned about your family and others with whom you live and work. Much of the book includes tips for all of the people on your team.

The recurring theme is to help you to be an increasingly active participant in your recovery. To reach the highest level of independence, you will want to:

1. Learn as much as you can about your medical condition.
2. Find out about the kind of care you will need—which doesn't mean you have to do everything by yourself.
3. Reach out to professionals who you can work with. Look also to people who have had experiences similar to yours to strengthen you.
4. Trust yourself. Work toward developing a positive attitude that can contribute to your healing.

This introduction is very similar to the conversation I

have with people when they leave the Rusk Institute.
I usually talk to the person whom I think of as the captain
of the team, together with the family.

In writing this, I thought about these conversations,
and the pride the rehabilitation team at Rusk feels when
someone we have worked with leaves us to return home to
resume their life.

Dr. Howard A. Rusk touched the lives of the three authors. I was trained in rehabilitation medicine by Dr.
Rusk. Florence Weiner's sister had her rehabilitation
training at the Rusk Institute following an accident. Dr.
Bell lived for twenty-five years in the Howard A. Rusk
Respiratory Unit of Goldwater Memorial Hospital, and
now lives in the community.

My coauthors join with me in wishing you well. If this
book is useful to you and your family, it will have served
its purpose well. We eagerly look forward to hearing whatever you would like to share with us.

> —MATHEW H. M. LEE, M.D., F.A.C.P.
> Medical Director
> The Howard A. Rusk Institute of
> Rehabilitation Medicine
> New York University Medical Center
> New York, New York

Introduction

Coming home from the hospital is the beginning of a journey—a trip that will last the rest of your life.

If you've ever taken a major trip, chances are you bought a tourist guidebook or two. For most of us, these comprehensive guidebooks are overwhelming in their attempt to cover every detail of possible interest to every type of traveler. But no two travelers are alike; each has a different itinerary. In much the same way, Dr. Howard A. Rusk, the founder of the Rusk Institute of Rehabilitation Medicine, believed in the unique needs of each person.

One way to read a tourist guide is to scan the entire book, returning to mark off the attractions that are of interest to you and that fit your budget of time and money. A travel agent can help you make certain decisions, but ultimately, no one knows you as well as *you*.

This book can be used in the same way. Think of the lists and charts as tourist maps which do not have to be used verbatim. As with all guidebooks, the most important sections are the marginal notations and personal observations of the traveler.

The health care professionals with whom you will be working are like your travel agent. They know more about the conditions than you do, but they cannot order you to do anything. You are the client.

Chances are that if you are reading this book, you have been in the hospital because of a heart attack, open-heart surgery, or another major cardiac procedure, or because you live with another type of heart condition.

Or you may be the wife, husband, daughter or son, or friend of someone hospitalized with a heart condition and want to learn more about what it takes to make life work again, and the nature of your role in the recovery process.

You and your family may understandably not be thinking about your recovery at home if you are still flat on your back in a hospital bed. So let this book be your guide to the positive challenges you may confront in all stages of the healing process.

It's possible to have major heart surgery and be back at work several weeks after the operation. That's the good news, and it's exhilarating. Being back at work should also mean the development of new and improved life-styles, including a more healthful diet, an exercise program, and stress reduction.

What you do at home in the time between leaving the hospital and returning to work can set the tone for the way you will live from now on. It is another chance to be healthy simply by doing what is good for you.

Whatever it is that you want to accomplish doesn't have to be done all at once or by yourself. In addition to health professionals who can help implement your life-style changes, you can call upon the members of your family, friends, or someone you employ to assist you as you regain your strength.

This book will point you in the direction of dozens of new allies and helpers, ranging from your doctors to nurses, physical therapists and occupational therapists, nutritionists, social workers and psychologists, to your primary helpers at home, along with new friends that you can meet at chapters of Mended Hearts, coronary care clubs, and cardiac exercise programs.

Once you're on your way to recovery, the right attitude

is essential in maintaining a proper and healthy course. One highly educated executive celebrated his return to work by ordering a double cheeseburger at lunch. Another intelligent, sophisticated young woman lit up a cigarette within moments of returning to her desk. It may seem foolish, but all of us, children and adults alike, think we fool ourselves and others with self-indulgences like these. Of course, we may believe we are getting away with something with this kind of behavior, but we're not.

The dozens of preventive and wellness-oriented strategies described in this book can work only when you develop a mind-set determinedly dedicated to your improved health. An added dividend to this type of thinking is the elation you'll feel because you can take credit for making it happen.

You can focus on different chapters as your needs change and you move from one recovery stage to the next. Initially, you and your family will want to know what questions to ask before you leave the hospital. You'll find the specific questions to ask the nurse about your care at home, and what to ask your doctor about possible reactions to medications. When you establish a relationship with a cardiologist, you'll want to know more about communicating effectively in order to maximize the time spent together during periodic office visits.

And while recovering at home, you might want an informal schedule to follow, as well as a chart to remind you when to take your medication. You may like to know how to conserve your energy in the things you do every day. Families will be interested in support services for caregivers, and organizations that can help you make the transition from hospital to home and from home to work. The people you live and work with will want to know the warning signs of a heart attack, how to get help in a hurry, and what to do in case of an emergency.

You and your partner may be concerned about intimacy after a heart attack or open-heart surgery and would like both assurance and more information.

It might be difficult to imagine now, but someday you and your family and friends will be thinking of taking a trip. When that time comes, you will be interested in the services that airlines provide for travelers with heart conditions.

No matter where you are on the road to recovery, simply start reading at the point in this book that discusses where you are now. Make your own notes in the margins, and make copies of the charts so you can use them for as long as you like. The following chapter summaries will help you on your journey:

Chapter One: Leaving the Hospital Here you'll find out what information you and your family will want to gather from the hospital staff. Included are suggested questions to ask your doctor, the nurses, physical therapists, and social workers, who will direct you and your family in the exciting process of returning home.

Chapter Two: Recovering at Home The staff of the Rusk Institute provides practical advice on how to plan your day and how to create an informal schedule; how to arrange your kitchen, bedroom, and bathroom so the clothes and utensils you use most are within easy reach for greater independence; and how to implement other energy-saving strategies. A chart with a suggested informal daily schedule is included, as is a place to record your blood pressure, medications, and comments to share with your doctor. In addition, there are tips from men and women with heart conditions on handling "homecoming blues."

Chapter Three: A Family Endeavor Families share their experiences and give advice on how to take care of your recovering family member. You will find a description of home care services, a discussion of the responsibilities of a personal care aide and a visiting nurse, and the cost of these services.

Chapter Four: Taking Charge of Your Health The Rusk cardiac rehabilitation medical team gives practical advice on how to find the best medical care, including ways to communicate effectively and to establish a sound partnership with your doctor. Included are suggested questions to ask about your medical condition, medications, and symptoms that need to be reported.

Chapter Five: Strategies for Living Tips, strategies, and suggestions from the Rusk rehabilitation specialists on how to put your program into action, including discussions about how to set goals and the professionals and peers who can help you maintain your program. Ways to incorporate exercise, eat properly, and handle stress are covered. Here, too, you will find reassurance and information about intimacy and heart conditions.

Chapter Six: Getting Back to Work How to handle the challenge of returning to work—whether to the same job or something new—with practical guidelines on finding a balance between work and the other parts of your life, plus tips on coping with job-related stress.

Chapter Seven: Being Safe The everyday role of the family in avoiding and handling an emergency, including specific steps to take in an emergency, and guidelines to determining the warning signs of a heart attack. Physical therapists and occupational therapists provide a room-by-room checklist for preventing home accidents.

Chapter Eight: Travel Tips on having fun while traveling, with information from experienced travelers with heart conditions.

Chapter Nine: Information, Services, and Products
Where to find the home care services in your community, and where to find support for caregiving families; how to locate personal care aides, physical therapists, and other professional services.

Each chapter ends with the actual words of a person who has experienced recovering at home with a heart condition.

How To Make the Most of This Book

• Purchase a school notebook or loose-leaf binder and arrange it by month, by subject, or any way that makes it easy to use according to your own personal style.

• Every time you come across an item that seems especially useful to you, enter the page number and topic in your notebook.

• You may also want to use a binder or folder to save bills and organize them into two categories: "Paid" and "Unpaid." Keep receipts from any health care–related purchases, contracts from home care agencies and suppliers, pertinent letters, and whatever else is important to save for your own records or for insurance and tax purposes.

• On page 199 you will find a place to list the telephone numbers of your doctors, personal care attendants, people at the hospital who will answer your questions once you're home, emergency numbers, and your insurance policy numbers. Make a copy for your notebook, or use the page in this book, and flag it for easy referral.

When people attempt to find help from health care

services, they can become discouraged by the seeming lack of services and impersonal attitudes on the part of people they encounter. Sometimes this can cause them to turn away from the worthwhile services that actually are available. There are, however, good and caring professionals whose work it is to fulfill the physical, psychological, and emotional needs of individuals and their families who are dealing with illness. You will know when you find them—keep on looking until you do.

Chapter One

Leaving the Hospital

Discovering the ways in
which you are exceptional,
the particular path you are
meant to follow, is your business
on this earth, whether you are
afflicted or not. It's just that
the search takes on a special urgency
when you realize that you are mortal.

—BERNIE SIEGEL, M.D.

F OR MANY PEOPLE, the experience of leaving a hospital is like graduating from school; it is accompanied by the same feelings of exhilaration, anticipation, and anxiety. All of these feelings are valid and, as with the challenges of any new beginning, the way to take control of your new situation is through action.

Choose someone, perhaps a family member or a friend, to serve as your hospital advocate. Keep your advocate apprised of everything; ask them to sit in on the talks you have with your doctor; have them there when you meet with the physical therapist. If you have had surgery, the nurses can give you and your advocate—as well as the rest of your family or other helpers—instructions about the postoperative care that you will need.

An advocate can call to make an appointment with the social services department, especially if you are going to ask them to make arrangements for a personal care aide or a nurse.

Most hospitals also have staff members who serve as patient representatives, and who can be very helpful in answering your questions.

Men and women who have left the hospital after a heart attack or bypass surgery say that if you don't get answers to all of your questions—for example, questions about your medications, exercise, and symptoms to report to your doctor—while in the hospital, you can continue when you are at home. You can always call your doctor with the questions that haven't yet been answered. Likewise, your family should think about the kind of information they will need to best care for you and help in your recovery. But no matter when or where you ask your questions, remember: Go slowly. Think about what you want to say to your doctor, the nurses, or any of the others on the hospital staff who have worked with you and who may have information that is useful. Try to get the answers you need without being intimidated by the staff or made to feel that you are bothering someone.

One way you and your family can stay organized is by keeping a notebook for the names, telephone numbers, and other information that you will be collecting. A combination datebook-notebook is especially handy for keeping track of notes, appointments, and frequently called telephone numbers.

TIPS FOR YOU AND YOUR FAMILY BEFORE LEAVING THE HOSPITAL

Here are some examples of the type of information the hospital staff can give you. If possible, these discussions should include you, your advocate, *and* another member of your family. Make sure that someone is appointed official note taker.

• Discuss with the appropriate doctors and nurses your most pressing problems. It helps to write down your questions in advance and then record the answers you get. You will probably have more questions after you leave the hospital. When they occur to you, write them down and ask them when you next see your doctor.

• Ask any questions that may help in your understanding of your medical condition, your surgery, and the results of your tests and other procedures that were performed. Ask the doctor's opinion of what you can expect as you recover. For examples of specific questions, see page 81.

• Ask what instructions you need for your care at home, particularly postoperative care.

• Ask for prescriptions for your medications, syringes, and any other medical equipment, such as a ventilator, oxygen therapy, or a walker. You will also need prescriptions if home nursing services and physical therapy have been ordered by your doctor. Some medical equipment and supplies are available in home health care stores and can be ordered by your pharmacist.

• Ask the nurses about items you need at home for your comfort and safety, such as a bathtub chair and a hand-held shower head. Many drugstores and home health care supply stores stock the items you want or can order them for you.

• If you are not given a written hospital discharge plan when you leave the hospital, ask for one. Hospital discharge plans vary but usually include a description of your condition, a list of all medications with complete instructions on their use, a diet, an exercise plan, a restricted-activities list, and, if needed, prescriptions for home nursing and physical therapy.

• Ask the nurses what you and your family need to know about your care at home, postoperative instructions, how to monitor your vital signs, and the symptoms that may arise that need to be reported to your doctor.

• Ask the hospital dietitian what you and your family need to know about your diet based on your doctor's recommendations. Ask for printed menus and recipes. For more about the services of nutritionists and how to locate one in your community, see page 176.

• Ask your doctor or the physical therapist to explain your exercise plan, how to take your pulse, and what your target heart rate should be during exercise. Ask your doctor if there is a supervised cardiac exercise program in the hospital or nearby.

• If home nursing services have been ordered and you would like the social worker to handle these arrangements for you, make an appointment with the social work department. But you are under no obligation to have the social worker order these services for you. You can make *your own* arrangements. In either case, check your insurance benefits and find out which home care agencies you must use.

• Ask your doctor, social worker, or patient representative to tell you how to obtain a copy of your medical records from the hospital.

• Ask for your next appointment with your surgeon, cardiologist, or your own doctor. Make an appointment that is convenient for you.

• Ask the surgeon, if you have had surgery, to send a report on your treatment to your cardiologist and your own doctor. Ask that a complete report of your hospitalization be sent to each of your doctors.

For suggested questions for your doctor, see page 81.

Specific Questions for the Nursing Staff

Family members can learn about the home care services that are necessary and those that are optional from the hospital nursing staff. The nurses can tell you about postoperative care, nursing procedures, and precautions you should be aware of. You can review how to take your pulse, how to monitor your blood pressure, and how often to take both readings.

Here are some commonly asked questions of the hospital nursing staff. Feel free to add others that you may have.

• Are there instructions about my medications, medical procedures, and home care in the hospital discharge plan that need to be explained? Are there complete instructions regarding diet, physical therapy, exercise plan, and any special equipment prescribed to me?

• Can you tell me the purpose of each of my medications, instructions on how they should be taken, and how to keep a schedule of the time they are taken? Are there any potential side effects?

• What should I know about postoperative care, including: incision care, possible signs of infection, signs of rejections (if an artificial organ or device has been implanted), heart rhythm problems, bleeding, skin care, exercise, monitoring blood pressure, and fluid retention? If the incision is still healing, are special supplies or instructions needed? Should the dressing changes be sterile? Are there signs of incision problems, such as redness or swelling, that we need to be aware of?

• Will pain medication be ordered by my doctor? Should this medication be taken at the earliest onset of pain? Are there special instructions, and what side effects are possible?

• What are the signs and symptoms we need to know that indicate an emergency?

• What activities, such as walking up stairs, must I avoid?

• What kind of pain should be reported to my doctor?

• Will a nurse and/or physical therapist come to my home? For what length of time?

• Will the nursing staff be available to answer my questions over the phone after I leave the hospital? If so, what are their name(s), telephone number(s), and extension(s)?

SPECIFIC QUESTIONS FOR PHYSICAL THERAPISTS

Based on the results of your exercise stress test, your doctor and a physical therapist will create an exercise plan that you are to follow.

If you are uncertain about how to monitor your pulse when exercising, or have other concerns that keep you from beginning the prescribed exercise plan, call your doctor rather than wait to ask your questions at your next appointment with your doctor.

For more about finding a physical therapist in your community, see page 176.

Here are some commonly asked questions of the physical therapists.

• What kind of exercise should I do when I first come home? How often should I exercise? For how long do I need to exercise, and at what intensity? What instructions does my family need to supervise the exercises?

• Are there detailed instructions about exercise in my written hospital discharge plan?

• What is my target heart rate? How is it calculated and what does it indicate? How do I take my pulse rate during exercise? How often should I take my pulse?

• If my doctor prescribes it, would I benefit from a cardiac rehabilitation exercise program? What are the advantages of this kind of program? Does this hospital or one close to my home have such a program?

• What about warming up before exercising and cooling down afterward?

• Which household work should I avoid, especially if I've had surgery? What about stairs?

• Will the physical therapy staff answer my questions after I leave the hospital? If so, what are their name(s), telephone number(s), and extension(s)?

The Social Work Department

Most social work departments at hospitals are understaffed, and many are not equipped to handle the large number of people who may leave the hospital in a given period of time. So if your doctor has ordered home nursing visits, you, your advocate, or a member of your family should call for an appointment if you would like the hospital's social work department to make these arrangements for you. Most social workers can order prescribed home nursing care, physical therapy, and medical equipment.

You have no obligation to purchase any home care services or medical equipment directly from the hospital, and the social work department can make these arrangements only with your permission. Any of the services and equipment offered by social workers may be obtained independently by you or a family member. For more about home care services, see page 175.

Having arrangements for home nursing care and physical therapy made for you by the hospital's social work department is convenient but may allow less opportunity for you to actively participate in the selection process. Instead, you and a family member may wish to interview and hire a personal care aide yourselves, either before you've entered the hospital so that the aide is available when you return home or after you're already home. (For more about finding a personal care aide, see page 175.) Remember that a nurse or physical therapist who has been prescribed by your doctor must come from a home care agency approved by your insurance plan.

Increasingly, many families decide to have a personal care aide on a part-time basis—especially if a family member is elderly or has had surgery.

Specific Questions for a Social Worker

• Are the home nursing visits and physical therapy prescribed by my doctor in my written hospital discharge plan?

• If we make our own arrangements for a personal care aide, can you recommend several home care agencies, or suggest other community resources?

• Does this hospital offer a supervised cardiac exercise program?

• Do you know where the Mended Hearts and coronary care support groups meet?

CHECKING YOUR BILL

Before leaving the hospital you are entitled to a full explanation of your hospital bill. If there are questions about the charges, a family member should make an appointment with the billing office to go over the bill.

There are a number of excellent organizations that can provide you with guidance about your bill. The People's Medical Society—462 Walnut Street, Allentown, PA 18102 (800-624-8773)—will send you a fact sheet about decoding your hospital bill, and what to do if you have been overcharged. They will also send a fact sheet on filing a complaint.

The American Association of Retired Persons—601 E Street NW, Washington, DC, 20049 (202-434-2277)—provides free help in deciphering bills and in dealing with insurers. To learn more about this organizations's informational and referral services, as well as discounts for members, see page 181.

The People's Medical Society, which is a consumer health-advocacy organization, recommends the following when you suspect an error or question a charge on a bill:

• Request an itemized bill. Contact your insurance company and request an audit of your account. Ask for a

Utilization Review. If you're a Medicare recipient, contact your nearest Social Security Administration office.

• Inform the hospital when you have not received a treatment or service for which you were charged.

• If the hospital threatens you with legal action directly or through a collection agency, and you have been charged for services you have not received, contact your state's Consumer Protection Agency office.

• If you are still unable to resolve your problem, you may want to consider retaining legal counsel.

A Checklist for You and Your Family

Before leaving the hospital, make sure each of the following points have been addressed:

• You've received a written discharge plan that lists your medications with complete instructions, your recommended diet and exercise plan, the prescribed home nursing services, physical therapy program, and restricted activities.

• Prescriptions for medications, home care services, physical therapy, and any necessary assistive devices, such as a walker, oxygen therapy, or other equipment, have been given to you.

• Most of your questions have been answered by your doctor, the nurses, a physical therapist, social worker, and dietitian.

• The names, telephone numbers, and extensions of the staff who said that they will answer your questions after you leave the hospital are written down in your notebook.

• You and your family have met with the social worker and understand the home care services available to you, the home care services prescribed, and your insurance coverage. You have given permission for arrangements to be made by the social worker for a nurse, physical therapist, or other home care service, or you have decided to make your own arrangements.

• You have checked all the charges on the hospital bill, and if there is an error, it has been adjusted.

• You have requested a complete copy of your hospital record.

• You know when your next appointment will be with each of your doctors, and have a tentative schedule of other appointments to follow.

From an interview with a sixty-three-year-old man who had triple-bypass surgery

It's not a matter of "making it" with a heart condition; it's more like, do you or do you not want survival? Do you want an everyday life or do you not? Yes, I want a life.

"... I am one among millions of people living with a heart condition ... I plan on staying around a long time, and living a full, marvelous, productive life."

I know I have heart disease, and the corrective surgery I had doesn't take it away. I don't feel less a person because of it, and I don't let depression enter my life-style. I'm not going to let this thing or anything beat me—I am one among millions of people living with a heart condition. In fact, I plan on staying around a long time and living a full, marvelous, productive life.

Thirteen years ago during my hospital stay, I was visited by a lady from Mended Hearts. Of course, I was somewhat fogged out because this was mere days after my surgery. All I heard her say was, "I had the same kind of surgery as you, and so have the people in our organization. If you need questions answered, or if your family has questions, we want to help." When I got back on my feet, and was well enough, I went to a few meetings. And then I started to visit people who were about to have open-heart surgery, or already had it.

Today, we're much more educated and we're better consumers than we were thirteen years ago. Now I'm very definite about what I expect from a doctor. After all, I'm paying. I don't want to be waltzed around, as I call it. I don't want my doctor to respond to my question of "How am I doing?" by saying, "Don't worry about anything." It's my body, and I want to know what I'm supposed to do to make it better.

Chapter Two

Recovering at Home

What lies behind us and what lies before us are tiny matters compared to what lies within us.

—Ralph Waldo Emerson

When You First Come Home from the Hospital

Coming home from the hospital can be both wonderful and overwhelming for everyone in the family. You may be fortunate to have a caring family, friends, neighbors, and others—including professionals—but being at home is not like the hospital, where the real world and its pressures are kept away. In your own home, life goes on all around you and insists that you be a participant.

When you first come home from the hospital, your main goal should be to allow your body, mind, and soul to heal and strengthen as much as possible. You need to try to find the right balance between too little activity and overexertion.

Some people have an encouraging support team of family and friends who manage to fulfill what is needed without experiencing either exhaustion or undue sacrifice. Others find that although their family members are willing, they simply lack the wherewithal to provide care. They may be ill themselves, emotionally overwhelmed, or elderly. Perhaps they live at a distance or are too committed to their work to have much time to spare.

Other reasons, not so obvious, are personal resentments, marital discord—which can be intensified during the crisis of illness—and psychological problems that make the support ineffectual. These feelings need to be expressed openly in order to be resolved.

Many families find that while women traditionally assume the lion's share of nursing care, they may also keep house, go to the bank and to the supermarket, prepare and serve meals, and hold a full-time or part-time job outside the home. For these and other reasons, families realize that when a family member is ill and professional home care is necessary, they must utilize whatever services will make life easier—especially now, given the growing policy of early hospital discharge. And if the services aren't covered by insurance and are costly, families find they must pay out of pocket for what is needed.

EVERYDAY LIVING

We start with the most basic activities: getting into and out of bed, dressing, bathing, preparing breakfast, walking around in the house, and then going outside.

It's best to get out of bed and dress every day. Complete bed rest actually deconditions the body: It lowers the heart's pumping capacity and reduces the capacity of the lungs, alters your heart rate and blood pressure, and increases your susceptibility to pneumonia. These metabolic changes may adversely affect the healing of heart muscles. Instead of remaining in bed during the day, you probably should rest and take short naps in a comfortable chair with your legs elevated, particularly after you eat or walk, or when you feel tired.

To get started in the morning, do some slow stretches before getting out of bed. Bend your knees and hips, then straighten them a few times; raise your arms overhead a few times or at a height comfortable for you, then lower them. Take a deep breath while you raise your legs or arms and exhale when you lower them.

To get up from bed, slowly raise your body from a lying to a sitting position. Make sure you feel strong enough to balance without getting dizzy or experiencing difficulty breathing. Continue to sit on the bed with your feet down for two or three minutes, then slowly get up and stand for a few seconds.

By moving slowly and not making abrupt changes in your position, you are less likely to become dizzy or faint. If you are straining in order to get to a sitting position in your bed, especially if you have had surgery and are in pain, it may be because your bed is too low or the mattress is so soft that it doesn't give you the leverage you need to maneuver.

This can be easily remedied. If the bed is too low, wooden blocks purchased from a lumberyard can be used to raise it. Telephone books or other large books can also be used, but make sure they are evenly balanced. If the mattress is too soft to give you the needed leverage to lift yourself easily to a sitting position, place plywood between the mattress and box spring for added firmness. When you want to watch television or read in bed, use a wedge pillow to support your back.

Try to have the bed near the bathroom, at least for the first few days at home. If at first you find that it is difficult to walk to the bathroom, or if the bathroom is far from the bedroom, use a commode chair. Don't be embarrassed about asking for assistance.

It's a good idea to keep an informal schedule, especially when you first come home. You will probably find that your regular routine takes longer to accomplish, and it's wise to take it slowly and rest as needed. Should you become extremely fatigued at any time, or have difficulty breathing, or are perspiring excessively, you may have overexerted yourself. Immediately stop what you're doing, and keep all activity to a minimum until you have regained your strength.

Try to notice when you feel especially tired during the day. It may be after bathing, eating, or simply walking around. These are the times to ask your family, or your personal care attendant, for assistance. You will be able to accomplish more by conserving your energy. As you learn to gauge your endurance, you'll be able to determine how much you can do on your own and what activities require assistance.

Getting dressed, taking a bath or shower, preparing

something to eat, and eating itself are not necessarily thought of as exercise, yet these activities can make you as tired as if you had walked a considerable distance, especially when you do not have your stamina back. It's important to balance light and heavy tasks, with time in between to sit down and relax.

Rather than return to bed when you relax or take a nap during the day, it's best to use a recliner or sit in a comfortable chair and prop your legs up on a hassock or on a chair facing you with a pillow on the seat. Your legs should be raised to avoid or reduce swelling of the ankles.

If you don't feel like sleeping, use the time after breakfast to relax and read the newspaper or make phone calls, watch television, or listen to the radio. After you have rested or when you have the energy, take a sponge bath or a regular bath or shower. After getting out of the bathtub or shower, put on a terry robe and rest in a chair. Wait a few minutes before getting dressed if you are tired, and proceed after you have relaxed.

It's a good idea to lay out your clothes the night before. Do as little reaching or bending down for clothing in the closet as possible; this can be extremely tiring. You'll also want to sit down while you get dressed. Choose comfortable, easy-to-put-on clothes, such as jogging suits, which may be worn outdoors as well as inside.

If you live in a house with more than one floor, going up and down the stairs can be very tiring, and your doctor may recommend that you limit the number of times you use the stairs when you first come home. You may want to hang a basket on a heavy cord from the bannister on the second floor, and lower it to the first floor to fill it with items you need upstairs. When you get upstairs pull the filled basket up, and lower it again to be refilled. Keep medications, an extra pair of eyeglasses, and other things you need on both floors, so you don't have to keep making trips in either direction to retrieve them.

You may want to jot down when you have discomfort or pain, and bring the record with you on your next visit to your doctor. Together you may find what are the activities or stressors that trigger the pain. Perhaps a change in the dosage of your medications is indicated. The doctor may be able to make recommendations, or tell you what others have done that has brought relief.

The chart on page 50 combines an informal schedule; a place to keep a record of your blood pressure, pulse, and medications; and a place for any comments you would like to record and discuss with your doctor. You can use this chart or develop one that better suits your needs.

ARRANGING THE HOUSE FOR SAFETY AND COMFORT

The Bathroom

When you brush your teeth, wash, or groom yourself, it takes less energy to sit than it does to stand. All you need is a stool or a sturdy folding chair in front of the sink. If you can't see the mirror when seated, prop up a small mirror at a height where you can see yourself. Place your toiletries on an easily accessed shelf so you can reach them without having to get up.

If you find it is difficult to sit down in the bathtub and then get up on your own, it's best to use a bath transfer bench that has a back and adjustable legs. This is a very handy device that allows you to sit on it right in the bathtub. If you prefer to shower, you can purchase a bath

Time	Informal Schedule	Blood Pressure	Pulse	Medicine	Comments
8:30 A.M.	Wake up; take a resting blood pressure, if possible. Medicine before and after breakfast; check off on medication chart				
9:00 A.M.	Breakfast; relax/read the newspaper/watch TV/make phone calls				
10:30 A.M.	Take a shower or a sponge bath; put on a terry robe, rest, then get dressed				
11:15 A.M.	Medicine, if any; check off on medication chart; rest/read the newspaper; make phone calls				
12:00 Noon	Walk or prepare lunch; relax; eat lunch; medicine, if any; check off on your chart				
2:00 P.M.	Relax; medicine; check off on chart; plan dinner				
4:00 P.M.	Talk a walk; take pulse afterward; make a note of it				
4:30 P.M.	Watch television/read the newspaper; make phone calls/see friends; have a snack; medicine, if any; check it off on your chart; write down time/medication				
6:00 P.M.	Eat dinner				
7:00 P.M.	Relax				
8:30 P.M.	Get ready for bed; take medicines before bed; check it off on your chart; bedtime				

chair that fits in an enclosed shower. Either way, you have the advantage of getting out of the bathtub on your own or more easily when you are assisted. Remember to adjust the legs or seat, depending on the model, to a comfortable height, but always let your feet touch the floor of the bathtub or shower. If you feel unsteady, use a seat belt or any kind of belt that makes you more secure.

We recommend installing a safety grab bar at the appropriate height for getting in and out of the tub or shower. Be sure to have the bolts reinforced into the wall stud rather than only the tile so that it can support your weight without coming loose. There are also safety grab bars that clamp on to the tub. A variety of safety grab bars can be found at hardware and housewares stores.

Use a hand-held shower head so you can safely test the water temperature, regulate the water pressure, and enjoy the pleasant massage action. This will also save you from having to raise your hands above your head to wash your hair. Choose warm water, not hot, which could cause you to become dizzy or faint. Use a long-handled bath sponge or brush to reach your feet and back without bending.

Both bath seats and hand-held shower heads can be ordered from a local pharmacy or from a store that carries home care supplies. Check the yellow pages for listings. Comparison shopping always saves you money, because there is usually a wide price range for similar items. Benches and chairs run from about $50 to as much as $200. Hand-held shower heads cost $30 to $75 or higher, depending on the features. The more expensive ones have a button to control water pressure, which produces a soothing massage effect.

Nonskid strips or a rubber mat on the bottom of the bathtub or shower can keep you from slipping. Place a rubber mat or rubber-backed bath mat to step onto on the floor outside the tub. Towels or thin mats may wrinkle and cause you to lose your footing.

Have someone put up extra hooks in the bathroom so you can have your clothes and a towel handy. Consider using a terry robe instead of toweling yourself dry. It takes less energy to put on a robe, and a robe keeps you comfortable and presentable if you decide not to dress right away.

At first, you may want to have someone stay with you in the bathroom or close by when you bathe. Another option is an inexpensive intercom, which can be found at stores such as Radio Shack. If you are in the bathroom and you need something, you can use the intercom to ask for assistance. Intercoms are often set up in the bedroom, bathroom, and kitchen, but every house is different. If your home has more than one floor, for example, you may want a more extensive intercom setup.

The Kitchen

Try to arrange the kitchen so that you can easily reach dishes, pans, and anything else you use often. To avoid bending or standing while preparing meals, use a stool with casters. AdaptABILITY, the mail-order company (a division of S&S Worldwide), markets a Roll-Around-Chair that supports 90 percent of your weight and is outfitted with an extra-large padded seat. Call 800-243-9232 for the company's catalog, which features the chair and a wide variety of other comfort products.

To save steps, use a rolling cart to take dishes to the sink or dishwasher, or to bring food to the table. It's best to sit at a table or a counter, rather than in bed, to eat your meals. When you are able, make breakfast, lunch, or snacks for yourself.

When you have an appointment in the morning, or you need to be out of the house at a certain time for any other reason, attempt to do as much preparation as possible the night before. Set the table and ready the utensils, pans, and any food that doesn't need refrigeration. If you plan everything in advance and leave yourself enough time to rest after eating, you'll feel less rushed. This can only help the recovery process.

Your family may decide to make up weekly menus or to prepare food for the freezer that can be popped into a microwave or conventional oven and be on the table virtually in minutes. When there is good and appetizing food in the house, you'll feel less deprived by any new diet restrictions, and it will be easier to stay with your regimen of healthful eating.

Most people could benefit from better food choices, or so the media tells us every day. Any of the vast number of fine cookbooks on the market can make a big difference in how you plan weekly menus, read labels, shop, stock your pantry and freezer, and learn innovative food preparation. For a list of some outstanding cookbooks, see pages 184–86.

If you do the food shopping, it will take less time and energy if you know what you need in advance and shop in stores that are familiar to you. Keep a pad handy in the kitchen to jot down food items and the things you need for the house, and always shop with a list.

It will help to use a shopping cart, one you can push without getting tired. Whatever items you buy in bulk—for example, kitty litter or detergent—have someone else carry, or have them delivered. Likewise, let someone else lift your heavy grocery bags for you. When possible, choose stores that deliver. If you must carry packages, balance them equally on each side of your body.

ENERGY SAVERS

• **Use phone and mail-order services.** These days, you can order just about anything you want by phone or mail and have it delivered in a reasonable period of time. Shop at stores that deliver so you needn't carry heavy packages.

• **Hire an errand runner.** For all your errands, it may be easier to hire someone for a day or once a week than to do them yourself. High school and college students can go shopping, do chores, or serve as companions on outings and visits to the doctor. Bulletin boards in supermarkets, churches, temples, libraries, and colleges are places to post such a job opportunity.

• **Avoid rush-hour traffic, if possible.** Schedule appointments to avoid peak-hour traffic. If traffic is unavoidable, use the time to practice relaxation breathing.

• **Don't wait in line.** When you make an appointment with the doctor, ask for the first appointment of the day. This way, you stand a better chance of spending less time in the waiting room.

• **Start the night before.** Prepare your to-do list for each day the night before. You may want to revise your list in the morning in response to how you are feeling, your energy level, and other priorities. Be prepared to renegotiate deadlines with yourself.

• **Sit rather than stand.** When possible, sit on a stool or folding chair while bathing, brushing your teeth, and washing dishes. Try to push or slide objects rather than

lift them. Use a lightweight tray table on wheels to save
yourself unnecessary walking and exertion.

• **Try not to lift or push anything heavy.** When you do
have to carry something or exert energy, always exhale
before doing so.

• **Cook for more than one meal.** When preparing meals,
refrigerate or freeze individual portions for later.

• **Plan your week's wardrobe.** Put what you will wear in
one place in the closet to avoid using energy searching for
the items, particularly when you're getting ready for work
or an appointment.

• **Avoid reaching and raising your arms above shoulder height.** Dressing, shampooing your hair, doing laundry, preparing meals, and other similar activities can be
tiring—but they can also be simplified. Ask for help when
needed. When your stamina level is low, space personal
activities such as bathing, shaving, or washing your hair
over several hours.

• **Wear loose-fitting clothes.** At home, especially during
early convalescence, choose comfortable, lightweight
clothes. Jogging pants, cotton knit shirts, and lightweight
jackets are easy to put on, they put less strain on you
during any activity, and they machine-wash and -dry. Try
slip-on shoes to avoid bending down. Choose clothing
with nonbinding elastic waistbands, Velcro fasteners, and
front closures.

• **Keep an eye on the weather.** Weather conditions can
influence your energy. Excessive heat, cold, or humidity
may cause shortness of breath. Dress accordingly, and be

prepared for weather changes during the day while you are at work or outside.

• **When climbing stairs, monitor your breathing pattern.** First, breathe in deeply through your nose. Next, exhale through pursed lips as you climb a couple of stairs. Stop, rest, and breathe deeply and slowly. Continue climbing two or three steps while you exhale. Stand still when inhaling. Hold on to the stair rails whenever possible for extra support.

• **Organize the things you use most often.** At home and at work, have the things you use most often—glasses, keys—close at hand, and avoid having to reach or bend for them.

• **Schedule a breather for yourself.** Whether you're at work or at home, take time out to relax by closing your eyes and putting your feet up. If your work is especially stressful, arrange for activities that are noncompetitive. Be on the lookout for your own overscheduling.

Getting Up When You're Feeling Down

"Homecoming blues" is the term cardiologists use to describe the feelings of sadness, loss, and depression after a heart attack or bypass surgery.

Give your doctor every opportunity to help you. Ask him or her how others in your situation have managed. If your doctor doesn't respond in ways that are comforting to you, seek help elsewhere. For example, you may want to see a therapist who is experienced in working with people who have experienced a medical crisis.

Consider the following:

• **Compare yourself only to yourself.** We each have an inner clock that produces a personal healing schedule. Physical and emotional healing takes place at its own tempo. No matter what the statistics indicate, you are entitled to go at your own pace.

• **Insist on being a contributing member of the family.** Don't let anyone take away your role in the family or relieve you of the responsibilities that you can handle.

• **It's usually best to be with people.** Try to stay around people who make you feel good about yourself, especially when you are feeling depressed. Try to get past the feelings that restrain you. Do whatever it takes to get rid of the blues.

• **Choose to share your feelings with someone you trust.** You may not be up to talking to people right now because you feel tired, angry, tentative, and sad. When you are ready, find a family member, a longtime friend, or newer acquaintances from cardiac exercise programs, coronary care clubs, and organizations such as Mended Hearts.

• **You can't prevent stressful things from happening in your life.** Very often, stressful experiences bring on depression. However, you can manage stress by thinking ahead, stepping outside the urgency of the situation, and learning to relax. These are important skills for maintaining your balance and for recovering quickly following a stressful incident or situation.

• **Do not leave time unstructured.** Arrange your schedule to include leisure activities along with your work, relaxation time with others and alone, and rest along with physical exertion.

• **Trust yourself.** Rely on your intuition and instinct. If you can count on yourself, you are more likely to move into an action mode rather than dwell on the problem.

• **You'll feel better when you're helpful to other people.** It's amazing how often healing comes through an awareness of others. Making a commitment to another person counters the inclination to become bitter and give up.

• **Anger is a natural reaction.** Instead of ignoring or denying your anger, use it as the fuel to ignite your determination to go forward.

From an interview with a sixty-seven-year-old man who had a triple-bypass operation

In the hospital, my own doctor, my surgeon, my cardiologist, and the staff doctors visited me every day. When I came home, my "medical staff" was my wife.

She was scared stiff and couldn't sleep at night from all the responsibility. A few days before, in the cardiac intensive care unit after surgery, all these tubes were coming out of me. Then, suddenly, your family is supposed to know how to manage like a hospital staff. From ten doctors a day seeing me in the hospital, I went to not one medically trained person at home.

> "No one prepared us for what we would need at home, except how to take medications."

How am I really supposed to know how to evaluate my own recovery, or if it's proceeding as well as I can expect? No one prepared us for what we would need at home, except how to take the medications. It would take only one nurse or social worker who could tell people before leaving the hospital how to make the transition, just to let people know what they're likely to need and where to find it in the community.

No matter how capable and well organized you are in your personal life up to that point, enough happens in the hospital to shake you and your family to the core. All your feelings are heightened in the crisis, and it's hard to think through the simplest thing—you feel extremely vulnerable. So we had a family meeting to figure out what we needed help with and decided to get it, whether it was covered by insurance or not.

We called in a visiting nurse; it cost $80 a visit, but it was worth it. I had picked up an infection in the hospital and didn't know it; I needed an antibiotic. One of my medications was giving me a lot of trouble, and the nurse called my doctor and reported it to him. When the dosage was changed, I could tolerate it. My doctor wrote an order for a laboratory technician to come by to my house to draw blood because the nurse told him that's what I needed. Suggestions were also made of which bathtub bench to buy, and my bed was raised so I could get out of bed on my own without pain. Without the nurse, I wouldn't have gotten those things, or would have had to wait two weeks until I saw my doctor again. She helped me with things I couldn't possibly have known about on my own, and significantly enhanced the speed and quality of my recovery.

Chapter Three

A Family Endeavor

God, grant me the serenity to accept the things I cannot change, the courage to change the things I can, and the wisdom to know the difference.

—SERENITY PRAYER

*Advice for Family Members
  from Men and Women with Heart Conditions*

About Home Care Services

Insurance Coverage for Home Care

Home Care Costs Vary

The Client Bill of Rights

Interview

W E ASKED MEN and women who had had a heart attack, a bypass, or other heart conditions what they find makes the transition from the hospital to home less turbulent and how their families and friends can help. Families and primary caregivers were asked, "How do you take care of a loved one?" Their shared experiences, tips, and advice make up this chapter.

"The only thing that makes sense about having a heart attack is that you realize how precious and precarious life is," said the wife of a man who had a heart attack. "You name it, and we've been through it and learned from it. Our lives have been changed by it, and many changes are for the better. My husband was a workaholic, extremely impatient with himself and everyone around him. After his heart attack, prolonged depression immobilized him. A cardiac rehab program that had exercise, meditation, and counseling from people who have a heart condition helped lift the depression. He continues to meditate, and it works for him, and he's got us all meditating."

"The best advice is to get the very best medical care you can find, and a doctor you have confidence in," says a woman who has had two heart attacks. "Then complement the quality medical care with professionals you trust to learn how to stick to a program of eating good food and exercise, to quit smoking, excessive drinking, or anything else that keeps you from being healthy. Shore up your confidence with psychological counseling, so you can deal with the strains of daily living."

"What you feel most of all when you are sick is loneliness, the feeling of being apart from the rest of the world and envious of everyone who is healthy," says a man who had bypass surgery.

"My family and friends are my glue," says a woman who had a valve replaced and a pacemaker implanted. "It's a big surprise to see who'll stand by you and who'll drop out. A man I work with, who had a heart attack several years ago that I never knew about, came through for me with encouragement that I will remember for the rest of my life."

Here is some other advice for men and women with heart conditions and their families.

ADVICE FOR FAMILY MEMBERS FROM MEN AND WOMEN WITH HEART CONDITIONS

• **The more you know, the more effective you can be.** When you understand your family member's medical condition, the more effective and in control of things you can be. If you know what triggers pain and causes extreme fatigue, you are better able to devise coping strategies.

• **Families are partners in the recovery.** Encourage your husband, wife, or parent to do whatever he or she is able to do. Make it clear that you are willing to help whenever it is needed. All of you will benefit from preplanning and conserving energy. If you lay out clothing the night before, for example, you save yourself much bending and reaching the next morning; and if you set the table for breakfast the night before, you save repeated trips back and forth.

• **Get enough rest.** Divide responsibilities with everyone in the family. Include children and grandchildren who can do the shopping and run errands. This enables them to contribute to the family and to feel a sense of participation.

If you are the only caregiver, consider getting the help of a student, a part-time personal care aide, or a housekeeper. Caregiving family members need to take time to do the things they like and value. Take the help of other family members when it is offered, and investigate services in your community that you might have overlooked.

• **Protect your back by learning how to lift properly.** Various booklets and magazine articles provide advice about the best ways to lift. Look for diagrams explaining how to lift someone properly when transferring them into and out of bed or the bath without straining your back.

• **Create an informal, flexible schedule.** Especially during the early days of convalescence, leave enough time for the family member to rest after eating, bathing, dressing, visits from friends, and other activities.

• **Prepare for all trips.** Family members can make a list of what you want to accomplish, along with anything else you need to remember. Find out if there are long distances to walk or stairs to climb. Give yourself extra time to avoid the pressure of needing to rush. Plan something pleasant to do, such as stopping for a cup of tea or a snack, if possible.

• **Family members need to talk about the changes that have taken place in their lives.** Stored-up resentments can surface with more forceful and hurtful words than are intended. When the caregivers feel overburdened but are able to talk about it, problems are more easily identified and the family can look for solutions.

• **Have an emergency plan that everyone in the family knows.** Start cardiopulmonary resuscitation (CPR) training by calling your local chapter of the American Heart Association and Red Cross for locations of CPR classes in your community.

• **Most people who have a heart attack and bypass surgery return to work.** If the partner who had been the wage earner must now remain at home while the other partner becomes the wage earner, the one who remains at home needs to assume the responsibilities of keeping house. A role reversal takes getting used to and also requires a willingness on the part of all concerned to adjust to different responsibilities.

• **The encouragement of friends makes a difference.** Most friends rally 'round when there is an illness. Sometimes, though, because of their own fear of illness, some friends withdraw. If your family values the friendship, see if you can talk it out together.

• **Family members are welcome to attend meetings of Mended Hearts and coronary care clubs.** Most of the meetings are open to family members. Some support groups are for caregivers; others are for men and women with heart conditions. Even if the member of your family who has a heart condition doesn't want to attend, family members may find they will get a lot out of what they learn, and share with other family members when they get home.

ABOUT HOME CARE SERVICES

Many families decide to hire someone to help them at home, especially in the early days after the hospital stay. This is essential if you have had surgery or if the primary caregiving members of the family are elderly and have their own medical problems. Or if you live alone, you may hire a personal care aide, housekeeper, or someone to shop and to accompany you to the doctor when a family member is not available.

Even if it is on a part-time basis and not covered by insurance, another helper can give family members a chance to rest and renew, or return to work.

It takes considerable time and effort to locate a person who is reliable, trustworthy, and pleasant. That is why many families turn to an agency for help with this task. On the other hand, if you plan to have personal care assistance for an extended period of time, the advantage of training and managing a person you recruit, with whom you establish a schedule and salary, without the restrictions of an agency, may outweigh the effort. Whatever source you use, carefully check in advance the references of whomever you employ.

Personal care aides from home care agencies will assist you in your personal care, such as getting in and out of bed, handing you medications, shopping, preparing and serving meals, and helping you with the exercises that have been prescribed.

Usually, the personal care aides from agencies assist only the person they are assigned to care for. They are not expected to prepare meals or do laundry or chores for other members of the family. The law in most states does not permit an aide to dispense medications, to change sterile dressings, to give injections, or to draw blood for tests. A personal care aide is supervised by a nurse and any other professionals from an agency who make home visits.

An integral part of a home care nursing visit is educating the family. The nurse is likely to make an evaluation and assessment of your condition, and will answer the family's questions about your condition, home care, medications, and any pain or discomfort you may be experiencing. The nurse will monitor your vital signs, check for fluid retention, and provide other postoperative care.

Some of the basic services that are provided by home care organizations are:

Medical and skilled nursing care

Therapies (physical, occupational, respiratory, speech, and intravenous drug therapy)

Nutrition or dietary services

Hospice services

Medical equipment, including oxygen tanks, portable ventilators, and telephone devices for monitoring pacemakers

Some agencies provide a wide range of services, including pharmacy and laboratory services, as well as offering assistive devices such as walkers and wheelchairs.

Personal care services are nonmedical services, such as assistance with bathing, dressing, preparing meals, and other personal needs.

INSURANCE COVERAGE FOR HOME CARE

Medicare and most medical insurance plans for home care services are restricted to people who are homebound and who require part-time or "intermittent" skilled nursing care and/or physical or speech therapy prescribed by their doctor. Also, these plans cover only a limited number of visits. This rules out coverage for around-the-clock home nursing, which is reimbursed only under very limited circumstances.

Medicare and many insurance plans do not cover nonmedical personal care or homemaker services, prescribed drugs, meals delivered to the home, blood transfusions, respiratory therapists, transportation services, or nutritional and dietary professional services.

Each employer-provided group health maintenance organization and private insurance plan has its own unique benefits and constraints. Some plans provide for nursing visits, hospital outpatient services, therapeutic services, and pharmaceuticals.

Home care services must be prescribed by a doctor and be accompanied by a written care plan, and must then be approved by your insurance company or agency. All home care, including physical therapy and speech therapy, must be supervised by a registered nurse from an approved agency.

HOME CARE COSTS VARY

The services provided by home care agencies vary in cost, depending on the region of the country and on the agency. Costs are usually higher outside of large metropolitan areas and in outlying rural areas.

Most home care agencies require that you sign an agreement or contract before services are provided. A contract commits you to pay for the services or authorizes the agency to bill your insurance company or Medicare.

Charges are usually based on a visit, although in some instances the services are billed on an hourly basis. The charges are generally the same for registered and licensed practical nurses and are billed on a per-visit basis.

An individual paying out of pocket for nursing services can pay over $100 a visit or less than $75, depending on the agency and part of the country. Professional visits of physical therapists and social workers generally cost about the same as those of nurses, although physical therapists in private practice charge less than agencies.

The costs for the services of personal care aides and homemakers vary, depending on the area of the country, the agency, and the responsibilities. Most agencies require a four-hour minimum for personal care aides, and set guidelines for their responsibilities.

The constraints that insurance places on services can prove to be baffling, yet there are people who can give you the information that will make it less so.

If your doctor prescribes nursing or physical therapy, for example, and your insurance will cover the services, you can find approved agencies in your community by asking the hospital social services department. You may prefer to call several home care agencies directly to compare prices. Your insurance representative should be able to give you a list of the agencies to use, or your doctor may be able to recommend an agency. For more about locating home care services in your community, see page 175.

THE CLIENT BILL OF RIGHTS

As a consumer you have the right to:

- receive considerate and respectful care in your home at all times;
- participate in the development of your plan of care, including an explanation of any services proposed, and of alternative services that may be available in the community;
- receive complete and written information on your

plan of care, including the name of the supervisor
responsible for your services;

- refuse medications and counseling, or other services, without fear of reprisal or discrimination;
- be fully informed of the consequences of all aspects of care, unless medically contraindicated, and the possible results of refusal of medical treatment, counseling, or other services;
- privacy and confidentiality about your health, social and financial circumstances, and what takes place in your home;
- know that all communications and records will be treated confidentially;
- expect that all home care personnel within the limits set by the plan of care will respond in good faith to your requests for assistance in the home;
- receive information on an agency's policies and procedures, including information on charges, qualifications of personnel, and discontinuation of service;
- request a change of caregiver;
- participate in the plan for discontinuation of services;
- receive home care as long as needed and available;
- have access upon request to all bills for service regardless of whether they are paid out of pocket or through other sources; and
- receive nursing supervision of home care aides, if medically related personal care is needed; the supervision shall be performed by a registered nurse.

From an interview with a fifty-five-year-old man who had a heart-valve replacement

The doctors and other professionals who have helped me the most since I got sick have in common that they add to my self-confidence, not make me feel more uncertain. They have a "calling," understand their purpose, and are willing to share what they know. It comes across that they respect me as a person, and that means a lot when you've had a setback.

"Great health care professionals don't just walk up to you ... finding them is an active process ..."

I think you sense very quickly when you find a nurse, physical therapist, social worker, or a personal attendant, whether they are going to be part of the solution, or will make more problems for you. Great health care professionals don't just walk up to you, though; finding them is an active process wherein you have to ask people who they recommend, and check out their credentials.

I lucked into finding a good doctor, a real person, who had firsthand experience because he had had a heart attack himself. He couldn't do for me what I needed to do for myself, but he hung in there with me. He knew what was getting to me, and he listened to me about my fears of resuming sexual activity. He encouraged me to get some counseling, and recommended a therapist he knew.

After him, one of the best things I've done for myself since this recovery process began is joining Mended Hearts. They have chapters all over the U.S. Almost all of the people had open-heart surgery. Most of the members have solved the problems that I was worried about. Now, after four years, I'm an old-timer!

For a support group to be good at all, you need to know it's a place you can be yourself. It's not necessary to feel you have to spill your guts there. In fact, you don't have to say a word, if that's what you want to do.

I wouldn't exactly say that all my concerns have gone away, but I feel I've been given a second chance at life, and it's very clear to me now what's important.

Chapter Four

Taking Charge of
Your Health

You can learn to follow
the inner self, the inner physician
that tells you where to go.
  Healing is simply attempting
to do more of those things
that bring joy and fewer of
those things that bring pain.

—O. CARL SIMONTON, M.D.

Taking Charge of Your Health

For some people, the goal is to mend, recuperate, and restore their bodies to a healthy condition that is as good as—or better than—before hospitalization.

For others, the goal is to adapt to new ways of living that for a short period—or perhaps for the rest of their lives—will be different from the way they lived before hospitalization. Perhaps the largest number of people with a heart condition are somewhere between these two situations. You have "graduated" from the hospital to your home, but you're still not well.

You quickly gather from talking to your doctor that the emphasis is on you and your continued willingness to substitute positive, healthful alternatives for past habits. You'll see a reduction in your serum cholesterol, blood pressure, weight, and blood sugar (if you have diabetes). These will head downward if you make exercise a priority, cut down significantly on fats, salt, and sugar, maintain close to your ideal weight, throw out your cigarettes, and learn ways to manage stress.

What does it take to bring about positive changes that affect the most basic ingredients of your health? How do you reestablish a balance when you feel enervated by physical and psychic wounds? How do you take charge of your health after a heart attack or heart surgery? Who are the people who can help? At the Rusk Institute of Rehabilitation Medicine, we believe strongly in the miraculous power learning everything you can about your condition brings, and the vital part that you play in your wellness. The more you know, the more likely you are to have a goal and to find people who can assist you in all the ways that are best for you.

Some of the major issues most people need to address after a medical condition has been diagnosed are:

- to learn what doctors and medical centers specialize in your particular condition so you can get the best possible medical care;
- to find out everything you can about your medical condition and the care you will need, so you can participate in the decisions that affect you. Reach out for support from professionals, your family, and other people with heart conditions;
- to gradually learn to become as self-sufficient as possible—without doing everything by yourself;
- to try to understand your feelings of fear, anger, loss, sadness, and depression with the help of your family, friends, and professionals.

GETTING THE BEST MEDICAL CARE

• **Have one doctor who centralizes your health care.** Have a primary care physician who coordinates your medications from each of the doctors who treat you.

• **Your family physician can refer you to a cardiologist.** If you do not have a heart specialist, your doctor or other specialist can refer you to a cardiologist. You may want to ask friends, someone with a heart condition, or other health care professionals for a recommendation.

• **Look for a board-certified cardiologist.** When considering a cardiologist, look for a board-certified professional on the staff of a medical center or hospital, preferably one affiliated with a medical school. Most board-certified cardiologists use the initials F.A.C.C. to signify membership as a Fellow of the American College of Cardiology, a professional association whose members must be board-certified. However, not all board-certified cardiologists choose to become members of this association, so nonmembership does not mean a doctor is any less qualified.

• **Check the doctor's credentials.** No matter where the recommendation comes from, you and your family can check a doctor's training, certification as a specialist, and membership in medical associations. Your local library should have the *American Medical Directory*, which lists all physicians in the country.

• **Do your part in establishing a partnership with your doctor.** The relationship with your doctor should be one in which you both talk and listen. Actively participate in all the decisions that are made about your treatment. If there is a conflict with your doctor or you can't work together, you may need to find another doctor. Before changing doctors, try to resolve any conflict about your care.

• **Look for a hospital-based or independent cardiac rehabilitation program.** You may want to consider participating in a cardiac exercise rehabilitation program, and also have a consultation with a staff member, such as a dietitian, a physical therapist, an occupational therapist, a social worker, or a psychotherapist to address your personal concerns. The assistance of these professionals can give you insight into your medical condition that may bring about positive changes.

• **Don't hesitate to get a second opinion.** Do not be inhibited by thinking that your doctor will be offended if you consult another doctor for an opinion. This is particularly important when a medical procedure or surgery has been recommended.

• **Give your dentist and other health care professionals a list of all of your medications.** If you have a heart condition with a valve involvement, you need to notify your doctor before you undergo a dental procedure, whether it is a simple cleaning, the filling of a cavity, or a surgical procedure. Your doctor will prescribe an antibiotic to reduce the risk of endocarditis, an infection of the heart's inner lining or valves.

GETTING THE MOST FROM AN OFFICE VISIT

An office visit gives you a chance to ask all the questions you may have, including those that have been answered but need to be repeated away from the hospital setting. It is an opportunity for you and your family to learn more about your condition, ongoing care, your medications, and any side effects and difficulties you are experiencing. It is also a time to talk about your concerns, and to set realistic, personal goals.

Most doctors are busy people with limited time for office consultations, so it's a good idea to figure out beforehand what you want to accomplish. Here are some strategies to consider:

• **Go to the doctor with a family member or friend who makes you feel at ease.** This helps you stay relaxed and focused, which can help you get what you want out of the visit. Write down questions, or keep them in your mind, and put the most important ones first. A list of suggested questions for the doctor is presented below. Your companion can write down the answers the doctor gives to your questions, and help remind you of things you wanted to discuss.

• **Try to keep daily records to chart your progress and to discuss it with your doctor.** Your doctor may recommend that you keep a record of your medications, side effects, blood pressure, pulse, diet, and exercise. It may also be extremely valuable to keep a diary of the times you experience angina so that you and your doctor will be able to see a pattern of what causes your pain.

• **If your doctor uses technical terms or abbreviations that you don't understand, ask for explanations.** If you don't understand, don't be embarrassed to ask!

• **You are entitled to copies of your medical records.** If you need to consult another doctor for a second opinion or if you need to change doctors, it can save time and money to have the information that is needed.

• **Bring some food and medication to tide you over.** Be prepared for the possibility of a long wait. Bring snacks—nutritious ones, of course. And be sure to bring any medicine you may need to take during this time.

SPECIFIC QUESTIONS FOR YOUR DOCTOR

While you are in the hospital or at your next appointment with your doctor outside the hospital, you can learn from the doctor more about your medical condition, the purpose of each medication, the nature of any ongoing treatment, and the changes in your condition that should be reported. If anything is unclear or confusing, ask to have it explained until you are certain you understand.

Here are some commonly asked questions:

Your Medical Condition

- Can you describe my medical condition? What can I expect in terms of recovering?
- What does my family need to know about my medical condition, medications, side effects, pain, and warning signs of cardiac problems?
- What postoperative instructions does my family need to know? Which activities must I avoid? For how long?
- What kind of pain and other symptoms should be reported to you?
- To which hospital do you recommend I go should an emergency occur? Which ambulance service do you recommend?
- What can you suggest for continued feelings of anxiety or depression? When can I hope for some improvement? What do you suggest for others that brings relief?
- When may I resume sexual activity? What do I need to know about the effect of my condition on sexual activity? If I experience problems, can you offer me support or recommend other professionals?
- When I return to work, will I need to modify my hours or any other work routines?
- Will you send a report and/or speak with my other doctors about my hospitalization, including details about my surgery, results of my tests and procedures, and medications you have prescribed?

Exercise

- From the results of my exercise test, do you recommend I exercise on my own? Should I be in a supervised cardiac exercise program?
- What should my heart rate limit be during exercise? How often should I exercise? What should a workout consist of? How often during exercise should I monitor my pulse?
- Why is checking my pulse and staying below my prescribed heart rate limit so important?
- Do you recommend wearing a portable heart rate monitor instead of checking my heart rate manually? Which one do you prefer?

More about exercise can be found on page 110.

Food

- What modifications do I need to make in my diet?
- Can you recommend nutritional programs that have helped others you treat?

For more about food, see page 103.

Medications

- What are the generic and brand names? What is each medication for, and what are the expected results?
- How much do I take at one time? How often do I take it?

- How should it be taken? With food? On an empty stomach?
- How soon should the medicine take effect? How long should I wait before calling if the medicine does not help?
- Which are the foods, vitamins, and alcoholic beverages to avoid?
- Which are the over-the-counter products that may not be used when taking the medicine? Why?
- May the amount be doubled if one dose is missed?
- If I feel better, should I stop taking the medicine?

Possible Side Effects

- What are the potential side effects or adverse reactions?
- What are the specific side effects that must be reported immediately?
- May I drive while taking this medicine?
- Does the medicine affect the pulse rate? What bearing does this have on monitoring the pulse when exercising?

TAKING CHARGE OF YOUR MEDICATIONS

More than 70 million Americans have one or more forms of heart or blood vessel disease, according to the National Center for Health Statistics. More than half of all the people being treated for a heart condition are given at least one drug, and many take three or more, some for a number of medical conditions.

Some medications need to be taken two or three times a day, others only with food to avoid stomach upset, and still others before meals on an empty stomach. To further complicate what already can be confusing, several pills may look exactly alike. It's not easy to remember to take the right medicine at the right time and in the right amount for the length of time prescribed, but you can find a system and make it work for you.

Americans spend about $6 billion each year for heart drugs alone. Almost 2 billion prescriptions are written in this country each year, and 50 percent do not produce the desired results, either because incomplete instructions are given, or because the instructions are forgotten or are not fully understood. The label may not include complete information concerning the name of the drug and how it should be taken (such as with or without food and in relation to other drugs). You should also learn about foods and alcoholic beverages that must be avoided while taking certain medications. Some drugs need to be refrigerated; others should be kept at room temperature.

Many over-the-counter products, particularly aspirin and products containing aspirin (such as Alka-Seltzer, Midol, cough medicines, and allergy products), can increase the anticoagulating potential of Coumadin and cause excessive bleeding. Products containing ibuprofen and indomethacin (such as Nuprin, Advil, Indocin, and Motrin) can also interact with anticoagulants. Some foods, vitamins, and alcoholic beverages can also interact with heart drugs and cause troublesome side effects.

To keep track of medications, the Rusk Institute recommends these general guidelines:

• **As a reminder to take a medication, plan to take them at the same time that you perform some other regular task, such as brushing your teeth.**

• **Try to take medicine on time, but a half hour early or late usually isn't going to upset things drastically.** If you are more than several hours late in taking medicine, ask your doctor if you should omit the dosage, or double it the next time.

• **Keep a record to manage medications.** A handy way to keep track of all the medicines you take is to keep a chart. You will find a sample chart on page 88. Write down any side effects. If you skip a dose, for whatever reason, place an X in the box to indicate a missed dose.

• **Bring your record with you to discuss with your doctor.** When you fill in the chart, or any other record you keep, take it along when you see your doctor.

• **Color-code your medicine containers.** If you are having trouble reading the labels, you might want to color-code the container, or identify them by touch. For example, wrap a rubber band around one medicine container and glue a piece of emery board to the top of another. Make a note on your chart of the code that you use.

• **Ask your pharmacist to use capital letters on the label.** The label may be easier to read if larger letters are used. Or use a marking pen to identify the container.

• **Try using a plastic seven-day pill organizer.** Containers are available that have compartments marked for morning, noon, night, and bedtime. You can find these containers in most pharmacies and in health food stores. They're available by mail from Bruce Medical Supply (800-225-8446) for less than $10.

• **An electronic medication pillbox gently beeps to remind you.** Medi-Track, for example, an electronic pillbox that can be set for any schedule, and gently signals when it is time for you to take a medication. It shows the day and time you last opened the box and even flashes to indicate if you missed a dose. Available at Eckerd, Walgreen, Revco, Sav-On, and other drugstores, it's also available by mail, from Wheaton Medical Technologies (800-654-5455). It costs about $30.

• **Wearing a wristwatch with an alarm** is another useful way to remind yourself to take medicine.

• **Keep a backup supply of medicine at work.** It's convenient, and can be extremely important, to keep a small supply of medicine at work or anywhere else you spend time away from home. If nitroglycerin has been prescribed, carry several tablets with you at all times. Keep a backup supply at work and in other places away from home. Nitroglycerin is effective for only about three months and must be replaced regularly. It may be helpful to date the container in which you keep the nitroglycerin tablets so you're aware of when to replace them. Warm weather can also affect the strength of nitroglycerin.

On the following page is a sample chart to record your medication schedule.

SELECTING A PHARMACY

Surveys show that when a prescription is to be filled, most people take it to the pharmacy closest to the doctor's office or to the one closest to where the person lives or works. Obviously, convenience is one of the factors to consider when choosing a pharmacist. There are also other factors.

88

A CHART FOR RECORDING YOUR MEDICATIONS

Month Of: _____

MEDICINE	Day	AMT	1	2	3	4	5	6	7	8	9	10	11	12	13	14	15	16	17	18	19	20	21	22	23	24	25	26	27	28	29	30	31

Morning / *Afternoon* / *Evening*

Instructions: Write in your medicine and the amount you are to take. Put in the day of the week in the box under the date. Place a check in the appropriate box after taking the medicine. Place an **X** in the box to indicate a missed scheduled dose.

• Are the prescriptions competitively priced? Does the pharmacy offer discounts?

• Can the pharmacist be reached easily by phone? When there is an emergency during the night, on a weekend, or during a holiday when the store is closed, what provisions are made to make medicine available? Does the store deliver?

• Does the pharmacist keep a record of all your prescription medicines, your nonprescription medicines, and any allergic reactions you may have to medicines? (Some states require that records be kept so that the pharmacist can give advice about medication uses and possible interactions. In other states, you still are responsible for knowing this information about each of your prescribed medicines.)

• Does the pharmacist offer to answer questions and give you instructions about the prescribed medicines?

• Does the store accept your prescription insurance plan?

• Can you use a credit card to charge your purchases?

You might decide to buy your medicine in a large quantity from a discount house or order it through the mail, especially if it is expensive, needs to be reordered repeatedly over a long period of time, or is not fully covered by insurance.

READING ABOUT YOUR MEDICATIONS

To supplement what you learn from your doctor and pharmacist, ask if there is any written information about your specific medicines that you can take home with you. The pharmacy may also have available at the counter various reference books or computerized drug information.

Pharmacists use the *United States Pharmacopoeia*, which is generally considered one of the most reliable resources for standards and information on prescribed drugs. It has monthly updates. One volume is specifically for consumers and provides comprehensive data about a medication, its purpose, how to take it, frequent and rare side effects, and interactions with other medications. It is available to be read at the counter in many pharmacies.

About Your Medicines, a consumer guide to the most commonly used prescription drugs, covers a medicine's proper use, side effects, and precautions concerning drug and food interactions. It contains a brand and generic name index. Sold in paperback for $7.95, it is published by the U.S. Pharmacopoeial Convention (USP).

About Your High Blood Pressure Medicines, also published by the U.S. Pharmacopoeial Convention, gives an easy-to-understand explanation of high blood pressure and the drugs used for its treatment. It costs $7.50.

The Handbook of Heart Drugs, A Consumer's Guide to Safe and Effective Use, by Dr. Martin Goldman, is published by Henry Holt and Company. The $12.95 paperback profiles more than ninety different kinds of heart medications, explains how heart drugs work, and offers practical ways to work with your doctor to find medications that will serve you best.

Complete Guide to Prescription and Non-Prescription Drugs, by Dr. H. Winter Griffin, is published by The Body

Press/Perigee. The $15.95 paperback provides information on five thousand brand-name and generic drugs in easy-to-read charts. Each chart includes the dosage and usage, possible adverse reactions or side effects, symptoms of overdose, warnings and precautions, and possible interaction with other drugs, food, and other substances.

PHONING YOUR DOCTOR

Especially after you first arrive home after the hospital, the primary communication link with your doctor is the telephone. In the past you probably called your doctor infrequently. Now you and your family may find the need to call more often.

When you leave a message, ask when you can expect to hear back from the doctor. Your call should be returned within a reasonable length of time. If necessary, call again to make sure your message was received.

Ask your doctor about the best time to call for non-emergency matters. Some doctors set aside early-morning hours to receive calls.

- Write down the questions you want answered and keep them in front of you. Jot down the answers to help you remember them. You'll feel calmer and more organized with your thoughts on paper.
- Keep telephone conversations as brief as possible, but make sure you accomplish the purpose of your call.
- When you call the doctor's office, try to speak to a nurse who can give you answers to some of your questions and refer others to the doctor.
- When a prescription is needed, give the doctor the phone number of your pharmacy or ask your pharma-

cist to call the doctor. If the prescription cannot be filled over the phone, arrange to have someone pick up the prescription from the doctor's office, deliver it to the pharmacist, wait for it to be filled, and then bring it to you.

- To be prepared for an emergency, write down the following information and keep it close to the phone so it can easily be located. Use large block letters so that you can read it even without your glasses.
- Your doctor's phone number.
- The 911 number or the number for Emergency Medical Service in your community.
- The hospital emergency number.
- The telephone numbers of people who you want notified in case of an emergency. (For more about how to handle an emergency, see Chapter 7, page 150.)

EVALUATING THE RELATIONSHIP WITH YOUR DOCTOR

While you were in the hospital you were cared for by many doctors. Now that you're at home, your relationship is probably with one or two doctors—perhaps your family physician and a cardiologist. Since you spend considerable time on the phone and in the offices of these doctors, your personal relationships with them are important. For this reason, it's a good idea to give some thought to how you are getting along with your doctor. Talk it over with your family and friends.

Your recovery will be hampered unless you have confidence in these relationships. Here are some questions you may want to consider asking yourself.

- Do I have confidence in the doctor?

- Do I believe the doctor is caring?
- Would I recommend the doctor? If yes, why? If not, why?
- Does the doctor listen attentively and grasp what I say?
- Does the doctor encourage me to ask questions? Do I understand the answers?
- Does the doctor give me enough time, or do I feel rushed?
- Am I encouraged to be fully involved in my care? Am I given all the information I need?
- Does the doctor encourage me to get a second opinion when a medical procedure or surgery is recommended, or if I am unsure about my treatment?

From an interview with a forty-eight-year-old woman who has had a valve replacement and a pacemaker implanted

I lost sixty pounds. You know how I did it? Watching the fat content of food, reading the labels. You have to do that after a valve replacement.

Women are new in being treated aggressively for heart disease. Look at me, I'm a good example. I'm only forty-eight, and I have a mechanical valve. I'm the sole support for myself, and the stress at my job is ungodly. Women didn't always have the kind of work, along with family responsibilities, that we have today.

"Attitude is 95 percent of the healing process."

Attitude is 95 percent of the healing process. I can see it in the support work when I go into the hospital with my Mended Hearts Club. The problems are not going to go away, and your job is to find out what you have to do and do it. Not that I'm saying it's easy. Everything doesn't run smoothly, either.

For example, I have a very good doctor. He's seen me through a lot. But I hadn't been feeling well for quite a while *after* the valve replacement and pacemaker implant. One day I came to his office and told him that I thought I should feel better than I do. He asked me, "Is there something you think I'm not doing that I should be doing?" And I said, "I don't know. I only know how I feel, and something isn't right." He said, "I have a file here on you that weighs five pounds, and everything checks out."

He decided to send me for another echocardiogram.

But I knew what the problem was all along. It was Lizzie Jane. That's what I call my pacemaker. But nobody wanted to believe me; they think I'm off my tree.

I called "pacemaker evaluation" because they can do an electrocardiogram over the phone. I get a readout once a month, and this time when I called I had been feeling nauseous. I asked the nurse how the pacemaker readout was, and she said, "The reading looks good, but if you're feeling sick to your stomach a lot of the time, the pacemaker may need to be adjusted." I called my doctor and I went into the hospital, where a technician checked it. It turned out Lizzie Jane needed a new battery. My insurance paid ten thousand bucks for a new one.

I guess I'm a piece of work. But what I've decided is that it's all up to me, and nobody is going to care about or knows as much about me as me.

Chapter Five

Strategies for Living

The fact that the mind rules
the body is, in spite of its
neglect by biology and medicine,
the most fundamental fact
which we know about
the process of life.

—FRANZ ALEXANDER, M.D.

Cardiac Rehabilitation

Setting Personal Goals

*Strategies for Turning Good Intentions
  into Healthy Eating*

Making Better Choices

Calculating the Fat Content of Food

The Foundation of an Exercise Program

Going the Distance

Strategies for Personal Goals

Taking Your Pulse

Countdown to Stop Smoking

Intimacy and Heart Conditions

Interview

CARDIAC REHABILITATION

Cardiac rehabilitation has been defined by the World Health Organization as "the sum of activities required to ensure cardiac patients the best possible physical, mental, and social conditions so that they may by their own efforts regain as normal as possible a place in the community and lead an active, productive life."

The first phase of cardiac rehabilitation starts early in the hospital, usually within twenty-four to forty-eight hours. It begins with the physical therapist helping you perform a series of passive range-of-motion exercises, and progresses over several days to having you sit next to your bed and moving on as soon as possible to slowly walking in the hall.

An important aspect of this phase are the talks with your doctor, the nurses, physical therapists, dietitians, and any social workers and psychologists who are involved in your care. You'll quickly gather from your talks that the emphasis is on *you* and *your* ability to change the numbers by reducing your risk factors, along with the benefits, of course, from technology and medications that repair and regulate the heart. Your doctor can talk specifically about what you can do to strengthen and restore yourself to minimize your risks.

The second phase of rehabilitation takes place after two or three weeks of at-home recuperation, at which time most people have recovered sufficiently to participate in a medically supervised outpatient exercise program in a hospital or rehabilitation center, or are able to walk close to home accompanied by an exercise partner.

Most medically supervised and monitored cardiac exercise programs call for three or four weekly group exercise sessions lasting about thirty minutes each; over time, they increase to sixty minutes. Programs generally run twelve weeks. Depending on the participant and the scope of the program, exercise sessions may be followed by talks about diet, smoking cessation, weight control, and stress-management techniques. An essential part of the program's philosophy should be to give men and women an opportunity to experience and understand the mind–body connection first-hand and use it to deal better with their heart condition, their pain, and their lives.

What is expected—in addition to significant life-style changes in diet and increased exercise—is a commitment to set aside time for daily relaxation techniques to reduce the ravages of stress. With psychological support from professionals and help from fellow participants with heart conditions, the dramatic shift in reversing heart disease, alleviating pain, and increasing the quality of life for those who stay with the program after leaving the training is extraordinary. For more about these programs, see the list of mind–body books on page 191. For audiocassettes designed for people with heart conditions who cannot attend the programs, see the list of audiotapes on page 192.

Insurance coverage for medically supervised cardiac rehabilitation programs varies considerably from state to state and company to company. Some policies cover only a limited number of outpatient sessions; others will pay for the entire twelve-week program. Check with your insurance company and the cardiac rehabilitation programs in your area to determine precisely what is and is not covered.

The third phase, or community phase, of cardiac rehabilitation typically commences when a medically supervised rehabilitation exercise program is no longer necessary. Many people opt to join a cardiac fitness exercise program at a Y, or at a fitness center.

Your challenge is to find the ongoing support to sustain the transition to eating healthfully, and to incorporate exercise into your already busy daily life. You'll also have to work on cutting out smoking and excessive drinking, and on tackling the problems of overwork and emotional strains on the job. Often, trusted professionals and the support from family, friends, and people who have had similar experiences will strengthen your resolve. Many people are reassured when they realize that they are not alone when they talk to men and women who have had a heart attack or bypass surgery, and that their fears are shared by others.

Becoming self-sufficient is a learning experience, measured by how well you feel as your body responds to the care you give it. As with any endeavor, it takes motivation, discipline, and a belief that *you* influence your general state of health.

Many men and women have found that the personal crisis of a heart attack forced them to consider what really matters in the grand scheme of life. "Often during all that you have endured, you realize that your life is yours," said a forty-five-year-old man who had bypass surgery. "It's not your family's or your doctor's. You are the only one who can determine how you will live your life."

SETTING PERSONAL GOALS

• **Quit smoking.** If you are a smoker, your risk of having a heart attack is double that of nonsmokers. The risk of sudden cardiac death is two to four times greater. Since smoking is both a physical and a psychological addiction, seek out professional programs and people who can support you in your efforts to not smoke again. By not smoking, you eliminate one of the most menacing health risks.

• **Try to reduce total serum cholesterol to under 200 mg/dl, with a total cholesterol/HDL ratio of approximately 3.5 or less.** For a cholesterol loss, decrease saturated fat to 10 percent or less of your total calories. In addition, eat more insoluble fiber, which is found in vegetables and whole grains, and maintain your recommended weight. Talk to your doctor or dietitian for specific recommendations about reducing fat intake and increasing your intake of fiber and whole grains.

• **Achieve a normal blood pressure of 140/90 or better.** The higher your blood pressure, the higher your risk of stroke, heart attack, and congestive heart failure. Blood pressure can be raised through inactivity, overweight, excessive salt intake, and increased stress.

• **Exercise regularly.** Physical activity lowers your risk of having a heart attack and raises your chances of survival after a heart attack. Aim to burn at least 150 to 300 calories each day by gradually increasing your walking or through other aerobic exercise.

• **Maintain blood-sugar levels.** Through a combination of weight reduction and regular exercise, the most common type of diabetes—type II, or non-insulin-dependent, diabetes—can be completely controlled or eliminated.

• **Maintain a body weight within 5 percent of the normal range.** Remaining close to your ideal weight reduces your risk of getting high blood pressure, high blood cholesterol, and type II diabetes. It also helps improve the performance of your cardiovascular system.

• **Find techniques to diminish the harm of stress.** Complement quality medical care with techniques that calm the mind and gladden the inner spirit: relaxation breathing, meditation, visualization, biofeedback, psychological counseling, mutual-help support groups, and prayer.

STRATEGIES FOR TURNING GOOD INTENTIONS INTO HEALTHY EATING

By now you are aware of the golden rules of healthful eating and weight loss: Use less fat in cooking and at the table; choose fresh fruits and vegetables over processed and fast foods; switch from whole to low-fat and nonfat milk, cheese, and yogurt; eat less meat and try more fish and dried beans for sources of protein. Check the labels of salad dressing, canned soup, crackers, bread, and cake for salt and fat, and watch your intake of sweeteners, additives, and preservatives.

So why aren't we all eating wisely? Partly it is because knowing what is best for us and doing it are two different matters. Change is hard won, even when we know that the food we eat can harm us.

Members of Mended Hearts and coronary care clubs tell us that the natural tendency of most people after a heart attack or bypass surgery is to begin by making radical life-style changes, especially in their diet. Instead, begin by looking at what you're doing right. It may take less of a major overhaul to achieve your goals than you imagine, and it is more likely you will stick with it if it is gradual.

Most families are likely to be willing to give up certain familiar foods if there are others offered in their place. Consider your options without changing everything at once. The family cook may start by preparing familiar recipes using more healthful ingredients. Instead of sautéing in fat, substitute fruit juice, low-sodium tomato juice, reduced-sodium soy sauce, or wine. Salad dressing, quick soups, and desserts can be made from the heart-healthy recipes found in the seemingly unlimited choice of cookbooks. For a list of some of the most outstanding heart-healthy cookbooks, see page 184.

Remember that not all substitutions are painful! For example, you can eat omelettes and other egg dishes if they're made with cholesterol substitutes and cooked without butter.

Here are strategies to handle some of the difficult situations you'll encounter to keep your eating habits on track.

• **Plan ahead.** One of the most important techniques for maintaining your program of eating heart-healthy foods is to plan ahead so you have good food available in every situation without feeling deprived. For example, you may know you have a problem staying with your eating plan when you eat out. Be selective in your choice of restaurants; look for restaurants that will cook to your specifications. Decide beforehand how you are going to handle the situation.

Many restaurants now indicate heart-healthy items (those with low cholesterol and little or no salt) on their menus. Some restaurants have had these items analyzed by Heartsmart Restaurants International of Scottsdale, Arizona, which permits them to label menu entries with a ♥, the Heartsmart symbol.

• **Anticipate problem areas.** You are less likely to give in to the whims of the moment and pressure from others if you think through what you can expect in any given situation. For example, before going to a special affair where you know there will be food that's not right for you, eat something ahead of time so you won't arrive feeling hungry and consequently overeat. Ask the waiter to serve the salad dressing on the side and to omit gravy and creamed sauces. Have it your way.

• **Picture yourself in a difficult situation and then visualize a positive outcome.** Produce a movie in your mind. See yourself handling the situation. Positive visualization techniques are useful for gaining control over potentially troublesome situations. In our lives, the effects of stress result not so much from what we do or what happens to us but from the way we respond to them.

• **Use simple relaxation breathing for "tuning out."** The best relaxation techniques involve making a conscious effort to stay aware of the body's signals and to stay ahead of distress. In the book *Your Maximum Mind*, Dr. Herbert Benson describes the basic steps to elicit the relaxation response.

Pick a focus word, phrase, image, or prayer. You may also choose to focus on your breathing. Sit quietly in a comfortable position. Close your eyes. Relax your muscles. Breathe slowly and naturally, and as you do, repeat your focus word or phrase as you exhale.

Assume a passive attitude. Do not worry about how well you are doing. When other thoughts come to mind, simply say to yourself, "Oh, well," and gently return to the repetition. Continue for ten to twenty minutes. Practice the technique once or twice daily.

"Most people struggle with judgements and expectations, with thoughts and anxieties," says Dr. Benson. "Once you habitually elicit the relaxation response, you feel less anxious. As you learn to be more accepting of yourself and what happens during meditation, your ability to accept and be flexible extends into other areas of life as well." For a list of relaxation and guided visualization tapes, see page 192.

• **Think of your eating plan as a continuous invest-ment instead of an on-again, off-again diet.** If you keep it predictable and consistent, and anticipate and plan strategies, you should have better control of your eating. Think of the people who would be inclined to encourage you. In addition, your local Y or community center may have helpful classes and exercise programs.

MAKING BETTER CHOICES

• **Substitute skim milk enriched with vitamins A and D for whole milk.** Almost 50 percent of the calories of whole milk are from fat; 38 percent of the calories in "2 percent" milk are from fat, and 26 percent of the calories in "1 percent" milk are from fat. There's only a trace of fat in skim milk. To ease the transition, go first to 2 percent, then 1 percent, and then nonfat.

• **Try to replace two meat dinners each week.** Have a pasta-and-vegetable dish or a seafood dish that can be eaten along with a filling grain. When you do eat meat, choose leaner cuts of beef, like top round, eye round, or leg of lamb. Pour off the fat that accumulates in the pan. Buy the *select* grade that has the least fat, followed by the *choice* grade. If you have questions about which cuts of meat have the least fat content, or about the labeling, storage, and handling of meat and poultry, call the U.S. Department of Agriculture's hotline—800-535-4555— where home economists will answer your questions.

• **Get to know your microwave.** You do not need to add fat when you cook in order to prevent foods from sticking. One of the pluses of microwave cooking is speed—which should encourage you to cook low-fat dishes in quantity. Make large batches of homemade chicken stock for rice pilafs, tomato sauce for pasta, and hearty soups. Cook stew, soups, and gravies ahead of time. If you chill them or put them in the freezer, the hardened fat can be easily removed before the dish is reheated.

• **Use a butter "replacement" on bread and for cooking.** Try apple butter and fruit spreads on bread, and use butter substitutes, such as Molly McButter and Butter Buds, sprinkled on potatoes and vegetables. Margarine is made from vegetable oil and has no cholesterol, but it has the same number of fat grams as butter. If you use margarine, buy one of the soft tub margarines that has a ratio of at least twice as much polyunsaturated fat to saturated. When cooking, use nonstick pans, and greatly reduce the amount of fat required for cooking. To sauté onions and garlic, start them in a tablespoon of olive oil in a nonstick pan, then add broth or water so they steam/sauté. Or eliminate the fat entirely and just use the liquid.

• **Pizza, barbecued chicken, and ribs are probably our most common take-out foods.** Except for the high quantity of cheese, pizza is a highly nutritious ready-to-eat food. Instead of cheese, ask for a topping of onions, broccoli, green peppers, and mushrooms. Remove the skin of barbecued chicken. Just say no to ribs!

Fast foods are high in fat and salt. Usually 40 to 55 percent of the calories come from fat.

• **Enjoy balsamic or raspberry vinegar or low-sodium mustard.** Use these condiments instead of salt to add zest to grilled fish, chicken, salads, and cooked vegetables.

• **Look for low-fat cheese that can be used in cooking.** Hoop cheese, often called "baker's cheese," is a soft cheese used in commercial baking. It contains less than a gram of fat and 10 milligrams of sodium per ounce. Use it in cooked dishes and serve it as a spread mixed with herbs. Try Sapsago cheese, a low-fat cheese, in place of Parmesan cheese, and skim-milk mozzarella instead of whole-milk. Remember to check the sodium content on low-fat cheese.

• **Make your own mock cream cheese.** Drain low-fat plain yogurt overnight in a strainer lined with cheese-cloth.

• **Instant hot cereals are higher in sodium than regular cereals.** Use regular Quaker Oats oatmeal and Cream of Wheat (or Rice) and other hot cereals unless they are flavored with sweeteners or are high in salt.

• **Insoluble fiber is beneficial for controlling weight and cholesterol levels.** Whole-grain breads, pears, pinto beans, wheat bran, graham crackers, blackberries, and strawberries are excellent sources of insoluble fiber.

• **Use concentrated frozen juices in cooking and baking.** Use unsweetened frozen juices in place of syrup on pancakes and waffles, and as sweeteners in cooking and baking.

• **Try grain beverages with the taste of coffee.** These are made of grains and chicory, with none of the caffeine. Most health food stores stock several brands. Some come in convenient packets that you can carry with you.

• **Try sparkling water or no-sodium seltzer with a twist of lime.** There are about 10 teaspoons of sugar in the average 12-ounce can of soda. A 12-ounce wine cooler has more alcohol in it than a 12-ounce can of beer. Sparkling waters and no-sodium seltzers are refreshing and healthy alternatives.

CALCULATING THE FAT CONTENT OF FOOD

Most food labels contain the calories per serving as well as the grams of carbohydrates, fat, and protein. To calculate the percentage of calories provided by fat, first convert the weight of fat in grams that is present in the serving to calories of fat.

The conversion factor is 9, meaning that 1 gram of fat contains 9 calories. In other words, 5 grams of fat in a serving would equal 45 calories (5 times 9).

If the total calories per serving is 120 and the fat per serving is 8, then 8 grams of fat per serving times 9 calories per gram equals 72 calories of fat. This means that 72 of the 120 calories are fat calories. To find the overall percentage, divide 72 calories by 120 total calories, which equals .60, or 60 percent.

If you want to know the percentage of fats without doing mental arithmetic, you can buy a nonelectronic calculator called the Percent-O-Fat Calculator that is available in health food stores for $5.95. If you can't find it in your health food store, call the manufacturer, APR Industries, at 800-266-3733.

THE FOUNDATION OF AN EXERCISE PROGRAM

An Exercise Prescription

Once you have completed an exercise test, the information from it is used to write your exercise prescription and to provide guidelines for work and recreational activities.

As in any written prescription, an exercise prescription is personal. Weekly energy expenditure during exercise depends largely on four factors, namely the type of exercise, frequency, intensity, and duration of your exercise session. You will be able to regulate all four factors.

You can remember the four key variables by thinking of the word "fit." It stands for *frequency* (how often you exercise); *intensity* (how strenuously you work); and *time* (how long you work), along with the *type* of exercise.

Aerobics is the exercise of choice for cardiac exercise training. Brisk walking, riding a bike, swimming, low-impact aerobics, aquatic aerobics jogging, and cross-country skiing are all aerobic exercises that start to burn fat at an early stage of the training session and ensure a constant supply of oxygen to the muscles. Aerobics literally means "with oxygen." To qualify as aerobics, an activity must be performed regularly, be rhythmic, involve the arms and legs, and be maintained long enough to increase the body's cardiovascular endurance.

Anaerobic, or "without oxygen," exercises are high-intensity activities performed for a short amount of time, such as sprinting, calisthenics, basketball, or tennis. In these activities, the muscles require more oxygen than your circulatory system can provide. As your breathing picks up rapidly, you feel "out of breath." At this point, you should stop exercising or slow down dramatically to sustain the intensity necessary to improve cardiovascular function.

Heavy lifting and isometric exercises are especially dangerous for someone with a heart condition, because they greatly increase blood pressure, decrease venous return, and increase the heart's workload.

If you have been inactive, have arthritis or another orthopedic condition, are extremely overweight, or have given up exercising in the past because of exhaustion, pain, or possible injury, begin by gradually incorporating additional activity into what you do every day. For instance, instead of driving, walk to work or to the store. If that's not practical, start by parking your car a few blocks farther than you normally would; or walk at a purposeful pace for five or ten minutes.

The level terrain and the climate control of indoor shopping malls make them favorite places for walkers and joggers in the early-morning hours before the stores open and attract shoppers. Increasingly, communities are sponsoring "Walk the Mall" programs.

Exercise with family or friends may provide social support and increased motivation.

Frequency

At the Rusk Institute we believe that people with heart conditions should ideally exercise at least three times a week. You will show a conditioning response, improved well-being and health, reduced tension, as well as significant cardiac benefits.

There is a proportional increase in orthopedic or overuse injuries in people who exercise at high intensities more than five days a week. Specific questions on exercise to ask your doctor can be found on page 83. The physical therapist in the hospital can also answer your questions.

Intensity

Your doctor will tell you at what intensity you should exercise. All of the numbers and the other specifics in this book are generalizations that vary according to each individual, as prescribed by your doctor and therapists.

If you monitor your pulse while exercising, you will be able to protect yourself simply by slowing down when you go beyond your range.

Time

In most supervised cardiac exercise programs, each exercise session lasts one hour, including warm-up and cooldown exercises. When you arrive at the exercise site, you and the other participants weigh yourselves, check your heart rate, and link up to the monitoring device.

The exercise session begins with at least ten minutes of warm-up exercise, such as stretching, light calisthenics, or perhaps walking. That brings each person's heart rate into the lower end of the target heart rate range. Thirty or more minutes of aerobic exercise within the target heart rate range will follow, and the session will conclude with at least another ten to fifteen minutes of cool-down exercises similar to those performed during warm-up. Each participant's heart rate and blood pressure is taken and recorded before leaving the facility.

When you exercise on your own you should follow the same basic routine.

Warm-Up Period

A warm-up consists of walking at a pace about seven to ten minutes below the training heart rate (that is, about halfway between your resting and training heart rates).

In cold weather, increase the length of your warm-up by five minutes to assure that there is an adequate blood supply to your heart and working muscles. If you have hypertension or if you experience cramping in your legs, walk seven to ten minutes in warm weather and an additional five minutes in cold weather.

Warming up starts channeling blood to working muscles and causes the heart and respiration rates to start a gradual rise; it also helps stiff muscles and joints to limber up.

To prevent injury, it is advisable to always warm up your muscles before stretching them. Stretching may also be done at the end of the exercise session, immediately after your cool-down.

Aerobic Exercise Period

Of course, the most beneficial portion of the exercise program for developing the heart and the circulatory system is the exercise session itself. Your workout should be continuous, and you should protect yourself by monitoring your training heart rate.

To gauge if you are working hard enough to accomplish your fitness goals and yet not so hard that your workout is unsafe, monitor your pulse and take the "talk test." If you are working out at a reasonable rate of aerobic exertion, you will be able to talk, although you will notice an increased rate of breathing and some perspiration. If you have difficulty talking, and your pulse indicates you have surpassed your target heart range, pull back until you reach your safe aerobic exertion rate.

Cool-Down Period

Just as the warm-up period is gradual, your cool-down period allows the heart rate and blood pressure to return to their resting states. Stopping suddenly may cause blood to pool in your legs and cause you to feel light-headed. In hot or humid weather, increase the length of your cool-down to assist your body in returning close to its resting levels.

Take your pulse to check your recovery heart rate after five minutes. If your heart rate is still above one hundred beats per minute, continue to walk slowly until it slows down.

Wait at least ten minutes to shower or bathe after exercise to allow all your body functions to return to a resting state. Keep the water at about body temperature, not excessively hot or cold. Water that is too hot slows the circulation and can cause dizziness; cold water can strain your heart.

Stretching

After each exercise session, include hamstring and calf stretches as part of your total body routine. You will have less muscle tension, and injuries are less likely to occur, because stretching prevents muscle strains.

Stretching promotes blood circulation and increases your range of motion, and is particularly beneficial after extensive bed rest.

It's important to make an effort to set aside eight to twenty minutes a day to stretch your arms and legs. Stretching is a good way to calm the mind and soothe the body.

Exercise and Weather Conditions

When it is hot, exercise during the cooler times of the day—the early morning or late evening. Heat stress can occur in conditions of high temperature, high humidity, and low wind, so exercise outdoors in a hot climate only if you are very fit and used to these conditions.

During the cold months, dress in layers so that clothing can be removed or put on as needed. Choose light clothes that are able to "breathe." Your first layer of clothing should be made of a material that wicks moisture away from the skin, such as polypropylene. Wool makes an excellent second layer. A lightweight water-repellent jacket is a good outer layer.

Keep layers loose in order to trap your body heat. The first thin layer removes perspiration from the skin, the second provides warmth, and the third protects against wind and rain. Some people like to wear a pair or two of simple cotton or wool socks. Others prefer a thin liner made of polypropylene, which wicks away sweat, under wool or synthetic socks. Wear a wool or synthetic cap or hood and mittens, which are warmer than gloves, to prevent excessive loss of body heat.

If you develop angina in cold weather, check with your doctor about exercising outdoors. You can protect yourself from cold air by wearing a ski mask or a scarf pulled loosely in front of your face. Breathing warm air will often reduce or prevent anginal attacks. If the day is windy, the first segment of the exercise session should be taken into the wind. This avoids excessive fatigue and chilling due to walking or running into the wind on the return trip.

GOING THE DISTANCE

• **Start gradually.** Attempt to build exercise into your schedule. Choose the kind of activities you enjoy, and stay with it even if at first you don't see marked results.

• **Choose the time that suits you best.** If you exercise as soon as you get up in the morning, you have the advantage of feeling well rested. If you exercise before you shower and dress for the day, it saves the energy of showering and changing clothes later on.

• **Your personal exercise prescription is unique.** Like anything that is prescribed, your exercise plan should be tailored to your specific needs. Based on the results of your exercise tolerance tests, your level of fitness, your particular condition, and your doctor's recommendations, it will tell you how often, at what intensity, and for how long you will need to exercise.

• **Stay within your prescribed limits.** Train regularly, without excessive peaks of activity. Avoid intensive competition. Never be out of breath or unable to carry on a conversation.

• **There are times not to exercise.** Do not exercise when you have a minor illness and a fever. After a minor illness, resume your exercise program cautiously. If you miss more than a week of exercise, cut your program back by one-third when you begin again. You lose fitness about twice as fast as it takes to build it up. Don't be concerned if you seem to be taking a long time to get back into shape after you have been out for a minor illness.

• **Wear a Medic Alert identification.** You can call 800-ID-ALERT, or write the Medic Alert Foundation at Turlock, California, 95381-1009. Most pharmacies have Medic Alert enrollment forms that you can fill in and mail. For more about the organization, see page 156.

• **To be on the safe side, always carry money for a phone call or for a bus or taxi should you become overtired while exercising.**

Week of: **EXERCISE PLAN**

MONDAY	TUESDAY
YOUR COMMENTS:	
PULSE: During Exercise After Cool-Down	PULSE: During Exercise After Cool-Down

WEDNESDAY	THURSDAY
PULSE: During Exercise After Cool-Down	PULSE: During Exercise After Cool-Down

FRIDAY	SATURDAY
PULSE: During Exercise After Cool-Down	PULSE: During Exercise After Cool-Down

SUNDAY	
	Target Heart Rate: _____
	Range: _____ _____
	Personal Goals:_____
	_____
	_____
PULSE: During Exercise After Cool-Down	_____

On the previous page is a suggested weekly exercise plan. If you make copies and fill it in, you can record your progress. Take your chart with you when you see your doctor so you can discuss your progress.

STRATEGIES FOR PERSONAL GOALS

Setting Goals

To reach your goals, it is a good idea to break them down into small pieces, then take the small pieces and use them as a bridge to the larger goals that may take longer to achieve. You might want to set as a goal your desire to exercise four times a week. Another goal may be to set aside a specific time in your schedule to exercise. In setting your goals, make them specific and measurable. Keep them realistic with guidelines from your doctor, physical therapist, or exercise physiologist. If one of your goals is to lose weight, find out if you have set out to accomplish this goal in a reasonable amount of time.

Your Personal Goals_____

_____

_____

Enlist the Support of Family and Friends

Enthusiasm is contagious, and it's pleasant to have someone along. At the start of your recovery, you will want to have someone with you when you walk. Later on, it's pleasant to have the companionship of an exercise partner.

List the people who can support you in exercising.

_____

_____

_____

Suspend All Self-Criticism

Make the time you exercise a gift that you give yourself. Feel pride in your accomplishments and trust yourself that you are giving your body what it needs in order to repair itself.

Record Your Progress

Keep track of how you are progressing. Also write down how you respond to the workout, particularly if you experience pain or excessive fatigue, and discuss this with your doctor. Photocopy the weekly exercise plan on page 117, or make a chart you prefer.

• **Learn your training heart rate.** By knowing the desired level of intensity of your workout, and by checking your pulse, you'll have a safe and effective means of monitoring your efforts.

   If you check your pulse and it is above your target heart rate, simply slow down.

• **Ask your doctor for guidelines for safe exercise.** Ask how long you should wait after eating before doing any strenuous exercise. Discuss the number of times you should work out each week, determine the appropriate intensity at which to exercise, and establish how long each exercise session should last.

• **Stop if you have angina.** Always take time out to rest if you have angina or other troublesome signs. Ask your doctor about the symptoms that may occur while exercising that you need to report at once.

• **Air pollution causes difficulty in breathing.** In extreme hot or cold and windy weather, and when there is smog or excessive pollution, walk indoors in a mall or in your home on a treadmill, or ride a stationary bike.

• **Drink plenty of water.** Even if you are not thirsty, your body needs fluids to avoid dehydration. Have a glass of water fifteen to twenty minutes before you exercise and drink small amounts of water—four to six ounces—at ten- to fifteen-minute intervals during exercise, especially if you are perspiring. Dehydration can cause an elevated heart rate. Continue to drink water after you've finished exercising.

• **Report symptoms to your doctor.** Notify your doctor if you experience any of the following during or right after exercise:

- angina
- light-headedness or dizziness
- nausea or vomiting
- leg cramps (claudication)
- breathlessness lasting more than ten minutes
- confusion or disorientation
- palpitations
- loss of color in the face or bluish skin tone

• abnormally high blood pressure

Symptoms that last at least a day also should be reported to your doctor, including:

• excessive fatigue that lasts at least a day and that continues even after you have slept
• difficulty in falling and staying asleep
• persistent racing heartbeat
• fluid retention accompanied by weight gain

TAKING YOUR PULSE

You can measure your own heartbeat by taking your pulse. The number of times you feel the pulse in a minute is your pulse rate. Your pulse rate is the same as your heart rate. When you take your pulse you can feel your artery give a little jump each time your heart beats.

Some people take their pulse before getting out of bed every day, before taking certain medications, and before, during, and after the cool-down of an exercise session. Ask your doctor when to measure your pulse, and whether to keep a record of your pulse rate.

• Using the pads (not fingertips) of your first two fingers, find your pulse at either the carotid artery (at the neck) or the radial artery (at the wrist).
• Press lightly until you find your pulse, especially at the carotid pulse, as pressure on this artery can sometimes slow the heart.
• Begin counting when the second hand of a clock or watch is at a point where a ten-second interval can be easily distinguished.

- Starting with the number 0 as a baseline, begin counting the number of heartbeats felt for a ten-second interval.
- Multiply this number by six to get your pulse rate for one minute.
- Take your pulse before, during, and after exercise to properly monitor your exercise.

If you have difficulty taking your pulse and you want to make sure you are maintaining your target heart rate, consider buying a watch that indicates your pulse. Casio makes a watch that indicates both blood pressure and pulse. Sporting goods stores usually stock this and other brands. It is also available through mail order from Self Care (800-345-3371) for $149.

Exercising is of greatest value when your heart rate stays within your safe "target zone"—high enough to stretch your capacity but not too high to be of concern. You can program your target zone into a heart-rate monitor that you wear on a comfortable chest belt over a T-shirt. It will beep if you go beyond your target zone. Electronic sensors accurately measure your actual heartbeat and you can see the results on an easy-to-read wireless wrist display. Check at sporting goods stores for a heart rate monitor, or call Self Care at 800-345-3371 to order the Polar Heart Monitor for $169.

COUNTDOWN TO STOP SMOKING

In his book, *The No-Nag, No Guilt, Do-It-Your-Own Way Guide to Quitting Smoking*, Dr. Tom Ferguson says that most nonsmokers simply do not know how best to help a health-concerned smoker. He suggests that "hard sell" approaches, which produce guilt and shame, are counterproductive.

The following guidelines for family and friends who wish to support a smoker's efforts to reduce their health risk are adapted from Dr. Ferguson's book:

• **Separate the smoker from the smoking.** Let your relative or friend know that you will continue to care about them no matter what they decide to do about their smoking.

• **Try to see the problem from the smoker's viewpoint.** If you attempt to look at how the person feels about smoking, it may help you to have a better understanding, and increase your tolerance. Smoking may be such a cherished part of someone's life pattern that smokers often feel to give it up would be like losing a good friend.

• **The temptation to simply ignore the negative health effects of smoking can be very strong.** The physical and psychological addiction can be so powerful that quitting can be painfully difficult. Smokers who do not have the courage to confront this dilemma deserve compassion and understanding, not ridicule and blame. A supportive relationship with a caring and understanding nonsmoking friend can make the smoker feel more secure and can provide the positive psychological motivation for change.

• **Encourage the smoker to do what they think is best.** Only when someone wants to do something about their smoking can progress occur. Instead of telling smokers what to do, encourage them to do what *they* think is best.

• **Suggest healthy, enjoyable activities.** Since engaging in sports is incompatible with smoking, and since activities such as concerts and religious services do not permit

COUNTDOWN TO STOP SMOKING

Week of:

	Write in Time	Place	Situation and Feelings	Rating 1–4	Alternatives to Smoking
MON.					
TUES.					
WED.					
THURS.					
FRI.					
SAT.					
SUN.					

Instructions: Make a photocopy of this chart and wrap it around your pack of cigarettes, holding it with a rubber band. If you unwrap the pack and smoke a cigarette, or take one offered by someone else, complete the information. Note the time, place, situation, and your feelings. Give each cigarette you smoke a rating: 1 is a cigarette you feel you can't do without; 2 is less necessary; 3 is a cigarette you could really do without; 4 is a cigarette you are not really sure about. This chart helps you to understand why and when you smoke and to create alternatives to smoking.

smoking, it may be helpful for the smoker friend or relative to accompany you.

• **You have rights as a nonsmoker.** You can ask your relatives and friends not to smoke in your presence or in your house or car, but you should do so in a polite, nonjudgmental way.

   Additional books to support you in not smoking are listed on pages 188–90.

The Countdown to Stop Smoking Chart is on the opposite page. You can make copies of it and wrap it around a pack of cigarettes.

INTIMACY AND HEART CONDITIONS

You are not alone if you feel anxious about resuming your sexual life. After a heart attack or heart surgery, men and women alike—as soon as they know they are alive—worry if it will ever be safe for them to engage in sexual activity.

   The concerns men and women have are only slightly different from one another. While a man may be troubled for varying periods of time by impotency and premature ejaculation, he also may have to adjust to more passive positions to place less strain on his arms and chest muscles and to conserve his energy. These positions might previously have been unacceptable, but they are now necessary to achieve intimacy and sexual satisfaction with his partner.

   A woman who has had a heart attack or heart surgery may react for a time with general sexual dysfunction, particularly in becoming aroused and in reaching orgasm. Women as well as men can be concerned about their attractiveness because of surgery scars or a pacemaker.

Even if no one brings up these concerns in an office visit, or if a doctor hesitates to ask probing questions for fear that talking about sexual intimacy will be perceived as an invasion of privacy, the problems still remain and can loom very large in the overall recovery.

If you and your partner have questions and concerns about sexuality that would take longer to answer than the usual time allotted for your visit, ask your doctor for another appointment specifically to talk about these matters. Before the appointment, write down what you would like to discuss. Talking to your doctor probably will be reassuring and helpful. If you or your partner are uncomfortable talking with the doctor, you might want to talk to a marriage and sexuality therapist.

"Your partner is just as scared as you," according to Barbara Faye Waxman, a disability consultant in sexuality, reproductive health, and family life rights. "This is not a time to stay silent. You are entitled to go at your own pace, but you need to let your partner know what that pace is.

"Resuming your sexual life is a very essential part of healing, and receiving love and giving love and expressing your sexuality are a very important part of feeling alive again. Test the waters first. The first thing you may want is to just touch and cuddle, and intercourse may be something for later on.

"Start by asking your doctor for information and for assurance, and then go further for the support that you can get from people who have heart conditions and are working through the same issues. The local chapters of Mended Hearts and coronary clubs are excellent resources."

In his book *Heart Illness and Intimacy: How Caring Relationships Aid Recovery*, Dr. Wayne Sotile, a psychologist and family and marriage therapist who works with men and women with heart conditions and their partners, answers some of the questions people have following a heart attack.

About the concern over the safety of sexual activity, Dr. Sotile says, "Although the sexual response cycle results in cardiovascular changes, the changes are not different from those experienced during regular exercise. The average heart rate during lovemaking is 117 beats per minute, while blood pressure increases to a maximum of 145/87 during a typical sexual encounter."

"Your sexual expression is an interplay between your own and your partner's most intimate, most vulnerable, and most wonderful layers of that inner sense of self that houses your unique and special gifts," Dr. Sotile says.

From an interview with the wife of a fifty-year-old man who had a heart attack

From a vantage point of five years since my husband's heart attack, I see some things I wasn't ready to accept at the time: He came closer to death than anyone would care to be, and his Type A personality significantly contributed to his having a heart attack. He gives everything he does one hundred and fifty percent, nothing less than perfection. The toughest job for him has been taking a hard look at his options, at how he was living his life and what he really wanted for himself.

The doctor told us that he was in relatively good health, with no complications and not too much damage. He could go back to work fairly soon. My husband was wondering if he would run his company again the way he used to, working eighteen-hour days every day. He has a pilot's license and flew all over the country, wherever he did business.

But after his heart attack, he started to live life scared. It wasn't depression, exactly; probably it was more like despair because he couldn't figure out where he was headed. There were times when he was either very quiet or seething with anger, mostly directed at me. Sexually, we were both too frightened to jump in.

> "It took us months before we could be at ease sexually . . . What we both wanted was to continue what we always had to prove to ourselves we had made it through."

Then, I remember it was my birthday and we got dressed up and went out to dinner. The waiter asked us if we wanted something to drink, and for a moment we paused. We weren't sure if it was okay. We sat there and looked at one another. You know how you laugh and cry at the same time? That's what happened to us. That night, we talked about what we were each feeling about the changes that had taken place. We told each other what we needed from one another. It took us months before we could be at ease sexually, but we touched and were intimate. We've always been very good partners, and intimacy is a very important dimension in our lives. What we both wanted was to continue what we always had to prove to ourselves we had made it through.

And about recovery on the more physical level, one day my husband got a call from the pilot who taught him to fly, someone who he admires. The pilot had heard about the heart attack and suggested that the two of them start walking together every morning at 6:30 A.M. Five years later, they still meet at 6:30 A.M., but now they don't walk, they run. Last year, they flew up to run in the Boston Marathon.

We keep a card tacked up on a board that someone sent my husband when he was in the hospital—something that Coach Vince Lombardi said—and it embodies our philosophy: "It's not whether you get knocked down. It's whether you get up again."

Chapter Six

Getting Back to Work

**What we must decide is
perhaps how we are valuable,
rather than how valuable we are.**

—EDGAR Z. FRIEDENBER

Considering Your Options

Looking at Your Work

A Plan for Returning to Work

Tips from People Who Have Returned to Work

Interview

Considering Your Options

"When will I be well enough to go back to work?" is one of the first questions most people ask their doctor after a heart attack or surgery. Typically, the answer given is based on your condition, how far advanced you are in your recovery, and the kind of work you do.

Your doctor may not have a complete picture of your work situation, how you respond to its pressures, and your apprehensions about keeping up when you return to work. You may be uncertain of your job security, whether you will be able to work for as long as you want, and if you will be able to meet your financial responsibilities.

Generally, men and women don't talk to their doctors about this personal upheaval or go into great detail about their jobs. The whole area of work and its stresses can go unnoticed, especially if the doctor sticks strictly to medical questions. Most doctors are hesitant to bring up personal subjects about work and financial concerns, fearing that it invades a person's privacy, as well as being out of their realm.

Yet most people find that their stress is job-related. You or a family member may need to initiate a discussion with your doctor about your concerns to explore the tensions that trigger upset and pain. Your doctor can tell you about what has helped other people in similar situations.

Millions of men and women successfully return to work after a heart attack and/or bypass surgery. Returning to work is an indication that you are handling another part of your life. Many people don't necessarily do the same work as before; old work habits may have to be revised in varying degrees. Some people are able to do some of their work at home part of the time. Computers, fax machines, and overnight delivery make this an increasingly popular option.

Work that requires heavy physical exertion, such as lifting heavy objects, that requires you to stand for long periods of time, or has you exposed to extreme heat or cold, is usually contraindicated.

For both physical and emotional reasons, it may not be possible to return to work. Age is also a consideration in your decision to continue to work or retire. It is possible that a reversal of the traditional work roles will take place in your family. A man formerly employed outside the home may be unable to find work and may need to assume the household duties, thus freeing his wife for employment. Any changes require patience, understanding, and a period of adjustment.

If your medical crisis has left you dwelling only on what you can no longer do, vocational counseling can give you a chance to consider new alternatives from which you can choose. Anyone who applies for disability benefits, whether their claims are approved or not, are considered eligible for services provided by their state's vocational rehabilitation agency. These agencies offer counseling programs and guidance, job training, and placement. Some states require a financial means test for vocational training, support services, and job placement. There are also private career counseling services.

Returning to work is as stress-producing as everything else you're facing. It is also an opportunity to ask yourself about what changes you need and want to make in your career. This may be a wonderful time to make a career change that will prove to be more satisfying than your old job.

In considering your present work or even a new and different career, list your physical capabilities and limitations. Factor in the return of your energy and endurance and what the impact will be on handling your work. Realistically evaluate your work, your commuting time, and the day-to-day stress factors.

Age can be a factor in the options. At this time in
your life, early retirement may be necessary. This can
cause hurt feelings when you're especially vulnerable.
Retirement may be viewed either as a punishment or
as a welcome reward for hard work. With newfound
time, you may find, as many people do, personal interests and hobbies that you were previously too busy to
pursue.

You also may want to consider a part-time job, either
the same type of work you were doing before or something new. If you are contemplating retirement, two
types of activities are especially important—continuing
education and working as a volunteer in a museum
or countless other places that welcome people with experience.

Many men and women who live with a heart condition
have found the choices open to them to be altogether
positive and unlimited in scope: taking courses, doing
volunteer work, perfecting a golf swing, traveling, or even
becoming self-employed and embarking on a second
career.

"I work and think differently about work now," a cre-
ative director for an advertising agency says two years
after a heart attack at the age of fifty-five. "Work used to
come before everything—my wife, my kids, everything—
in fact everything that really matters, but it doesn't any-
more," he says. "And I was the one who was doing it to
myself. I also ran out of excuses for not having time to
exercise, to eat right, or to quit smoking."

Making a personal plan in advance, before returning to
the job you held, finding out about your alternatives in
the hours you will be working, and, in general, exploring
new possibilities in your work options not only cuts
down on aimless worry but also prepares you for your
employer's concerns about your health as it relates to
your job.

Looking at Your Work

Here are some things to consider:

- Can I do the work I once did? Is it possible for me to return to the same job?
- What do I need now to do my work? Do I need to rest more frequently?
- Can I work either part-time or full-time? Can I work at home?
- Should I do another, less demanding kind of work even if I am paid less?
- If my work entails standing for long periods of time, can I instead work sitting down?
- What transportation can I use to get to work?
- What are my financial resources? Do I have enough to cover my needs on a long-term basis if I am unable at first to have the same earning power?
- What am I entitled to get in unemployment insurance and disability benefits?
- Do I need to think about moving closer to my place of work?
- If I move to a less expensive place, can I significantly reduce my expenses? What are the advantages and disadvantages of living somewhere else? Is it worth it to me financially and emotionally?
- Do I need to think about a shared living arrangement to reduce my expenses, to bring in additional income, or to create a feeling of added security?
- How do I want to spend my time? Do I want to spend my time differently than I did up to now? What are the interests that I'd like to pursue?

- What do the other people in my family or who I live with want to do regarding the shifts in my work life?

A Plan for Returning to Work

Try out your own plan—or, rather, the parts of it you can—a few times before you actually return to work to see how well you do.

Prepare as much as possible the week before you return to work. Then, after you are actually back at work, give yourself at least two weeks to evaluate the success of your plan. See what else you can do to modify your plan to make it even more effective. Ask yourself if you need to allow more time to rest or if there is a better way to get to work. As your strength increases, you'll be better able to know how to gauge your tolerance level and limitations as they relate to working.

Every year, thousands of people return to work after a heart attack or other medical condition. You may not know it, but several of your coworkers probably have similar medical conditions.

Do as much as possible the night before so there will be less to do in the morning:

- Put out your clothes to save time and energy.
- Plan your breakfast and set the table.
- Prepare lunch if you plan to take it to work.
- Provide yourself with healthful snacks to eat during the day. Take with you, or buy on the way, fruit, yogurt, or cut-up vegetables from a salad bar.
- Wake up early enough to give yourself time to rest and avoid rushing.
- Think about how long it takes to get ready and out the

door in the morning. Allow enough time when you begin to work again.

- Decide how you will get to work. Arrange to join a car pool, have someone drive you, use a private car service in your community, or take mass transportation.
- When you return to work, if you find that working an entire day is too taxing, see if it is possible to work part-time or fewer days; if necessary, in the earliest phase of your return, ask permission to come in later and leave earlier to avoid the rush hours.
- Your employers may overestimate you. You probably are reluctant to admit to any limitation for fear of putting your job in jeopardy, but if you overdo it, the consequences could be that you may need to stop working altogether. It's best to communicate clearly what it is you can and cannot do.
- Is there a refrigerator in your workplace? Perhaps you can use it to keep a supply of skim milk, yogurt, vegetables, and other foods, or medications that require refrigeration.
- Obtain a medical identification necklace or bracelet that lists your condition and medications. Be sure to wear it every day.
- Even if your family is protective of you, ask that they encourage you to try out new things as you seek alternatives to past work routines.
- Make every effort to become as self-sufficient as possible without doing everything yourself. You are entitled to ask for the help that you need to accomplish your goals.
- If you decide not to return to your former position or if you plan to make a job change, visit your previous boss or employer. They may know of other job openings that you could consider.
- It is against the law for an employer to ask about your

health until after employment is offered. If you have been discriminated against, you are entitled to file a complaint.

- Start reading up on the jobs in your area and in your particular industry.
- Find out about the employment agencies specializing in the work you do and check the help wanted ads in your local newspaper and in publications specializing in jobs in your field.
- Contact your state vocational rehabilitation agency. There are district offices in many major cities. They provide job counseling, job training, and placement based on your particular experience, skills, and the work you can do. Some states require a financial means test for vocational training, support services, and job placement.
- Look into colleges in your community that may offer career guidance.
- The number for the Social Security Nationwide Toll-Free Telephone Service is 800-SSA-1213. Call the toll-free number to learn your social security benefits. You may be entitled to supplemental security income or disability benefits. They will send you free literature on retirement benefits, disability benefits, Medicare, and survivor benefits.
- For information about your employment rights, transportation, accessibility, and accommodations to support you at work, call your local Independent Living Center. For more about the centers, see page 174.

The American Disabilities Act protects the rights of employees with disabilities. If you believe you have been discriminated against, contact the Office of Equal Opportunity.

Tips from People Who Have Returned to Work

• **Be flexible.** Think of new ways to make changes in the way you work. (Can you work shorter hours, work less intensely, and so on?)

• **Pace yourself.** Take time out to rest. Stick to regular, consistent hours, without extending it to overtime.

• **Take your medicines on time, especially if you're busy.** Keep backup medications at work. Make taking care of yourself a priority.

• **Communicate clearly about what you need at work.** If you have a tendency to take on everything and do it all yourself, get some assistance. For example, arrange for someone to drive you to and from work, join a car pool, or arrange for private transportation. Bring your own lunch or have it delivered. Be specific when you order so that you get it just the way you want.

• **Be a part of the activities at work.** Expressing your interest in people you work with promotes a sense of belonging.

• **Some people will treat you differently when you return to work because of their own insecurities about illness.** This can add another obstacle to returning to work. Try not to let it upset you too much. Use humor or a light attitude when dealing with the particular person.

• **Take short breaks.** Take time to rest and renew yourself. Learn some relaxation techniques. See page 191 for a list of books and audiotapes on meditation and other stress-reducing techniques. Try this: Breathe gently, then exhale slowly through your mouth. Pay attention only to your breathing and block everything else out. Get up and move to another place in the room (even if it's only in your imagination). Talk to yourself in a positive, encouraging way.

• **Consider professional psychological counseling or vocational counseling.** It may put into perspective some of your concerns about work. Chapters of Mended Hearts have speakers who talk about work-related problems.

• **If you are continually upset by your supervisor, see how the person deals with others.** You may not be the only target, and perceiving that will help you take the assaults less personally. Think of ways you can improve the situation for yourself.

• **Trust your own judgment about setting your own limits.** You are the only one who knows what works best for you.

• **Have a life after work.** If your work is stressful, plan noncompetitive leisure sports and relaxing activities when you are not at work.

From an interview with a forty-nine-year-old man who had a heart attack

Heart disease chased me my whole life. It was on my mother's side of the family, my grandfather had it, my father has it, and I just turned forty-eight when I got it.

In the late sixties, I moved out to California and went to law school at night. I practiced law until computers interested me more. The next dozen years I took three companies public, was a two-pack-a-day smoker, and drank more than enough. After fifteen years of marriage, with two teenagers, my wife and I separated. I wasn't proud of that. I missed my wife and my kids, and couldn't figure out where I belonged.

Last year, in the middle of a meeting, I got shooting pains first in my shoulder, then in my chest, and I started to sweat. An ambulance got me to the emergency room in time to have a heart attack. That really got my attention!

Two weeks out of the hospital, I go to see the cardiologist, and I'm still not feeling wonderful. I'm scared. I'm sad. Part of me wants to go back to work, but I'm thinking if I go back and keep working like I do, and get another attack, this time I won't make it. The doctor knows I've plenty on my mind. He listens to me and tells me that we'll work together. That made a big difference to me.

First he wants me to write down the things that drive me bananas. Present or past, anything I want to put in. "Pretend you're a reporter covering the story of how you live," he tells me. "For now, except for no smoking ever, don't make major changes." I start to write down what I eat, the exercise, and the things that are eating me up. The first thing I see is that with my schedule, there's no time to exercise. I know I have a short fuse, and I've got to do something about it.

> "I go back to work, but differently—I have reordered my priorities, with more time devoted to taking care of me."

I decide to go to a cardiac rehab program. First my insurance won't cover it, then they do. I stick with it because of the terrific staff, and I set aside a time when I exercise. A dietitian gives some classes in nutrition. I can handle the food with more planning. I start seeing a shrink. My wife and I get back together. I go back to work, but differently—I have reordered my priorities, with more time devoted to taking care of me.

Somebody at work gave me a little sign for my desk that says, "There must be something more to life than having everything."

Chapter Seven

Being Safe

Attitude makes all the difference.
Be not afraid of life. Believe that
life is worth living, and your belief
will help create the fact.

—WILLIAM JAMES

What Families Need to Know

Warning Signs of a Heart Attack

*The Pain of Angina Is Different
    from That of a Heart Attack*

How Family Members Can Help in an Emergency

Emergency Medical Service (EMS)

Calling Emergency Medical Service

How Your Doctor Can Help in an Emergency

Some Emergency Safeguards

*Where You Can Learn
    Cardiopulmonary Resuscitation (CPR)*

Emergency Medical Identification

Personal Alert Emergency Systems

Making Your Home Safe

Interview

WHAT FAMILIES NEED TO KNOW

When a member of the family has a heart condition, it means that everyone in the family must learn more about the medical aspects. Family members must learn about the pain experienced by another person so they can judge when to call the doctor, and when to utilize rest and relaxation techniques. Understanding the illness makes families capable of doing something that will make a difference.

Knowledge is essential in the event of an emergency. When you know how to be prepared for an emergency, and the steps to take to get immediate medical care, you increase the chances for your loved one to get immediate emergency medical care.

A person who suffers a cardiac arrest outside a hospital has a 25 to 30 percent chance of surviving. If cardiopulmonary resuscitation (CPR) isn't started until an emergency medical team arrives, the survival rate is just 5 percent. Family members may rationalize that their husband, wife, or parent has a good doctor so they needn't concern themselves about what to do in case an emergency occurs. What actually can happen is that an emergency can come without warning—and seconds count in a cardiac emergency. You may be the only rescuer at the time of an emergency, and you must know what to do—and do it—before the emergency medical service arrives.

Cardiologists maintain that it is imperative for families to be able to recognize the warning signs of an impending heart attack, to know what to do in a cardiac emergency, and to learn cardiopulmonary resuscitation (CPR).

The vital lifesaving skill of cardiopulmonary resuscitation (CPR) cannot preserve life indefinitely, but it can keep a person alive until more effective medical intervention is available to restore normal heart function. The new clot-dissolving drugs used to treat a heart attack can have a major impact on survival if administered promptly.

A good way to begin is for family members to talk to the cardiologist or primary care physician about the specific symptoms and emergency signs of the medical condition, about the possible reactions from prescribed medications that need to be reported, and the different kinds of pain that may be experienced. If there has been bypass surgery, you must know about the signs and symptoms that need to be reported to your doctor immediately.

WARNING SIGNS OF A HEART ATTACK

The cardiac rehabilitation staff at the Rusk Institute offers these guidelines to families. During a heart attack, most people have one or more of the following symptoms:

- Discomfort or a steady, squeezing pressure, ranging from an ache to a crushing or a burning sensation. The pain sometimes radiates from the center of the chest down one (usually the left) or both arms and to the shoulders, neck, jaw, or back.
- Gasping, difficulty in breathing, and/or shortness of breath.
- Sensation of heart palpitations or an irregular heartbeat.

In addition, the following symptoms may accompany the pain:
- difficulty in breathing or palpitations
- heavy perspiration

- sudden dizziness, light-headedness, and/or fainting
- nausea or vomiting (heart attack symptoms are often mistaken for indigestion)
- pale or bluish skin and lips
- cool skin and/or clamminess
- a sense of anxiety or impending doom
- shock
- unconsciousness

Unlike angina, the pain associated with a heart attack does not diminish with rest and it might last thirty minutes or longer.

Never delay getting help just to see if the attack abates by itself—even if the stricken family member resists getting help.

THE PAIN OF ANGINA IS DIFFERENT FROM THAT OF A HEART ATTACK

Angina attacks often occur during or following strenuous physical exertion, intercourse, a heavy meal, periods of intense fear, anger, or emotional stress, exposure to cold, or overeating.

Angina, *unlike* the pain from a heart attack, is usually relieved by rest and medication, usually nitroglycerin.

Angina has also been described as a feeling more like heaviness than pain. It can be accompanied by anxiety and frightening feelings of impending doom.

The pain of angina is frequently described as a tight grip or a squeezing cramp, a crushing feeling usually felt in the center of the chest, radiating to the left shoulder and arm. It may be accompanied by shortness of breath, profuse sweating, nausea, vomiting, palpitations, and/or fainting.

Your doctor can tell you how to space the dosage of your nitroglycerin or other medication, how much to take, and how long to wait if there is no relief from anginal pain.

How Family Members Can Help in an Emergency

- Focus on what you can do.
- Though you may be frightened, do everything in a steady and reassuring manner. The person will read your face and will react if you have panic in your eyes or in your voice.
- You may grasp the situation more fully than the person who is experiencing pain. If you suspect a cardiac emergency, get help *immediately* even if your family member wants to wait.
- Trust your ability to handle everything.
- Tell yourself that you can't panic.
- Reassure yourself that you are doing your best and you *will* be able to help.

Emergency Medical Service (EMS)

In more than half of the country you can dial 911 in an emergency and get help, according to the American Red Cross. By dialing 911, you can reach the Emergency Medical Service (EMS), the fire department, and the police.

Some communities do not have a 911 emergency telephone system. Telephone books have a listing of all the emergency services in a community. It it important to have this number handy.

If you are uncertain of the number for emergency medical services in an emergency, dial "0" and the operator will connect you to the emergency medical services. In many parts of the country, you can reach 911 from pay phones without inserting a coin.

CALLING EMERGENCY MEDICAL SERVICE (EMS)

• You contact the EMS by dialing the number in your community. When you report that you suspect a heart attack, you will be connected to an EMS dispatcher who will ask you your address.

• Give your exact location. If you are at home, give your street address, the cross streets, and the number of your house (or apartment house and apartment). If you are at work, give the building and the floor.

• Give the telephone number from which you are calling and your name.

• At night, turn on an outside light; if possible, send someone out to watch for the EMS and to direct the rescue personnel. Usually, at least two EMS personnel arrive with equipment.

• Try to stay calm, and answer the questions you are asked in clear, brief sentences.

• Be prepared to give the EMS technicians, as well as the doctors in the hospital, the names of all prescribed medications, the physical condition, and the telephone number of your doctor.

How Your Doctor Can Help In an Emergency

The doctor's answering service can locate him or her or can contact the doctor covering the practice. Even if it is a weekend or after hours, don't assume that the doctor will be unavailable in an emergency. Notify the doctor, but if you suspect that you or someone is having a heart attack or other cardiac trouble, get to the hospital without delay.

• **Ask your doctor for the steps to take in an emergency.** When you next see your doctor, ask when you need to get to the hospital or to call the EMS without waiting for the doctor's return call. Find out the location of the hospital nearest to your home that has twenty-four-hour cardiac emergency service, as well as one near where you work. Perhaps your doctor can help you work out an emergency plan.

• **Ask your doctor the symptoms that indicate an emergency.** Find out the specific information that you and your family need to give the EMS and the hospital.

• **Ask your doctor about other safeguards you should consider.** Particularly if you are alone for long periods of time, find out if your doctor recommends that you consider a personal response system to alert the EMS. Ask your doctor if you should become a member of Medic Alert. For information about personal alert emergency security systems, see page 156.

SOME EMERGENCY SAFEGUARDS

The Rusk Institute cardiac rehabilitation team recommends these safeguards to family members.

• **Be able to identify the early signs of a heart attack and other cardiac emergencies.** If a family member has recently undergone surgery or a medical procedure, has congestive heart failure or any other heart condition, has a pacemaker, or has had a transplant, ask your doctor for the warning signs you need to know that may indicate a heart attack or other emergency.

• **Know what to do in an emergency.** Write down the steps you need to follow in an emergency from what you have learned from your doctor and your cardiac resuscitation (CPR) course.

• **Act immediately.** If your family member is experiencing the signs of a heart attack—*and the warning signs last two minutes or longer*—make every effort to reach the doctor but do not delay getting to the hospital.

• **Expect a "denial" from your family member.** It's normal for someone with chest discomfort to deny the possibility of something as serious as a heart attack because they are frightened. *Don't let this stop you.* Take prompt action anyway. Most people wait close to two hours before calling their doctor or getting to the hospital for the medical care that they need.

• **Learn CPR.** Perform it, if necessary.

• **Know the locations of the hospitals nearest your home with twenty-four-hour emergency cardiac care.**

• **Keep a list of emergency rescue numbers next to the telephone and carry a copy with you.** In addition, make sure everyone in the family knows where the numbers are kept. Carry a copy in a wallet or purse. See the chart on page 199.

• **Carry a list of all medications with you.** In addition, make sure everyone in the family carries an up-to-date list of medications for emergency personnel.

• **Learn about Medic Alert.** This organization can assist you in an emergency by giving information to the Emergency Medical Service and the hospital. For more about Medic Alert, see page 156.

• **Make every effort to remain reassuring.** After EMS has been called, and you are waiting for medical help to arrive, make every effort to remain calm and reassuring. Make the person comfortable by loosening clothing, such as by opening a collar or a belt. It may actually be better for the person to be sitting rather than lying down in case vomiting occurs. Except for some water, it is best not to allow the person to drink anything.

WHERE YOU CAN LEARN CARDIOPULMONARY RESUSCITATION (CPR)

Local chapters of the American Red Cross and many Ys and community centers give a nine-hour hands-on course in CPR that allows you to learn and practice your skills on a specially designed mannequin, with supervision from an instructor. Generally, the course is given either in one day or in three-hour sessions one day a week for three weeks.

Many Ys and community centers offer basic CPR instruction. Your local chapter of the American Heart Association can refer you to a class in your community.

EMERGENCY MEDICAL IDENTIFICATION

Five million Americans are treated in hospital emergency rooms every year. A doctor you've probably never met before will have only a few minutes to make important decisions about the care you need. That doctor must have accurate information quickly about your medical conditions, precisely which medications you take, and those to which you are allergic.

Emergency medical professionals recommend the following:

• Wear a universally recognized emblem around the wrist or neck that can be custom engraved with information about your medical conditions.

• Look for a service that gives its medical staff twenty-four-hour telephone access to your computerized medical records.

• Be sure the service can store and quickly retrieve your vital medical information and the telephone numbers of your doctors and *two* people you designate to be called in an emergency.

• Don't rely on carrying only a wallet card. Emergency personnel often don't have time, or are not allowed, to search your purse or wallet. They are trained to look for an alerting emblem on your wrist or neck. Put on an emergency medical identification bracelet or neck chain and don't take it off. It could save your life.

Medic Alert Foundation International provides emergency medical information quickly and accurately to emergency personnel via a twenty-four-hour toll-free telephone hotline. The organization maintains computerized records on an individual's medical conditions, medications, and the telephone numbers of your doctor and two people you have designated to be called in case of an emergency.

Medic Alert also maintains an international implant registry for all types of implants, including heart valve prostheses and pacemakers. A newsletter and updates of recalls and new research is sent to members, doctors, and hospitals.

A Medic Alert basic lifetime membership is $35, a tax-deductible medical expense. The fee includes emergency hotline service, a custom-engraved stainless steel wrist or neck emblem with chain attached (sterling- and gold-plated emblems are slightly more expensive), and a wallet-card copy of all computerized information. Write Medic Alert Foundation, Turlock, California 95381-1009, or call 800-ID-ALERT. Most pharmacies have Medic Alert enrollment forms that you can fill in and mail.

PERSONAL ALERT EMERGENCY SYSTEMS

You may have seen a personal alert emergency system advertised on television or in a newspaper that is now being used by close to half a million people to bring immediate emergency medical service.

The system consists of a small push-button device, typically worn comfortably around the neck or carried in a pocket, that can be activated by a hand squeeze to send a signal to a monitoring center through a transmitter unit attached to the telephone. An operator will try calling the user back when the signal is received. If no one answers, or answers and reports that a crisis exists, a call is placed to the Emergency Medical Service and the doctor.

These home alert systems go by a variety of names, such as Lifeline, Lifewatch, and Lifecall. Lifeline, the first such system available to the public, currently has more than 100,000 subscribers.

Costs for the subscriber's initial equipment for the many systems available throughout the country vary from $300 to $900, with monthly service costs generally ranging from $10 to $20. To find out what systems are available in your area, call the hospital discharge office and the Area Agency on Aging. Be sure to thoroughly investigate any system you may consider buying for its effectiveness and total cost. Contact the Better Business Bureau to check if they have had any complaints about the company.

The National Rehabilitation Information Center (800-346-2742) will send you a listing of most of the personal security systems available. See pages 178–79 for more about the services offered by this organization.

MAKING YOUR HOME SAFE

Some of the things that contribute to home accidents after hospitalization are:

- the aftereffects of surgery and illness

- medications that alter vision, perception, cognition, and sensory distortions that can affect balance, judgment, recognition, and comprehension
- fatigue

Two-thirds of all falls in the home occur at the floor level and are the result of someone tripping over an object or slipping on a wet surface—particularly on a tile floor after bathing. Falls rank as the number-one cause of accidental home fatalities, particularly among people over sixty-five. Home accidents account for more injuries than motor vehicle and workplace accidents *combined*.

The National Safety Council estimates that close to 4 million disabling injuries each year are due to home accidents.

At the Rusk Institute, we recommend that a family member make a room-to-room check using the following guidelines.

Bathroom

- Install and reinforce grab bars for stepping up or down in the bathtub and where support is needed for negotiating turns.
- Put nonskid adhesive strips or rubber matting on the floor of the tub.
- Use mats with nonskid backing.
- Find a sturdy bathtub chair.
- Add a high-rise seat to the toilet, if necessary.
- Identify and mark medications, especially when several are prescribed.
- Make sure the bathroom is adequately lighted, with a regular light or a night-light that remains on throughout the night.

- Install an intercom for greater independence in the bathroom or for communication to any other room.
- Make sure there is a clear, well-lighted path to the bathroom at night.

Kitchen

- If you prefer to be seated while preparing food, can you reach over the stove burners safely? Be careful when wearing clothing with loose-fitting sleeves; they may drag over a burner and catch fire.
- Are the utensils, food, plates, glasses, silverware, and storage areas within your reach? Can shelves be lowered to accommodate these items?
- Is there a night-light that remains on throughout the night in case you go into the kitchen during the night?
- Regularly check the batteries of all smoke alarms throughout the house on birthdays or other easily remembered events. Install a smoke alarm outside the kitchen.

Bedroom

- Can you reach clothing in closets and on high shelves without losing your balance?
- Is there a night-light or a flashlight you could keep on a table to light your way if you need to get up during the night?
- Do your scatter rugs have a nonskid backing?
- If oxygen and ventilators are being used, each family member and any personal care attendant should know how to operate the equipment and understand what to do if the safety alarm sounds. The name and

telephone number of the vendor should be placed on the equipment or by the phone in case immediate attention is needed. Smoking should be forbidden near this equipment.

Halls/Stairs

- Are the stairs kept clear and well-lighted, and are there handrails on all staircases?
- Are the first and last steps marked? Hazardous changes in floor levels should be clearly marked with white or reflecting tape.
- Handrails should be able to hold a person's weight. They should be anchored into the wall studs and not into drywall or plaster.

Outside the House

- Are the curbs, gravel driveways, and sidewalks broken or uneven, posing potential hazards?
- Are there handrails on the staircases outside the house?
- Do the outside stairs need to be ramped?
- Keep the walkways free of snow and ice. Hire someone to shovel, if necessary.

From an interview with a sixty-year-old man who had two heart attacks

This kind of thing doesn't just happen—it's a long time in coming. But then when I didn't have a feeling of well-being, I knew something was haywire.

Since I'm a chaplain in a hospital, one day I decided to go to one of the doctors on staff, and asked for an in-depth physical. When the doctor finished, he said, "You're in good shape, your blood pressure is fine, your weight is fine, but let's do a cardiovascular workup to be sure."

The doctor looked at the results from the printout of the treadmill test and said, "You're about to have a heart attack." Then he gave me some nitroglycerin and sent me home. That night I had a strange feeling, took some nitro, and the next morning I went back down to the cardiologist to relay what had happened. Right there, I had another episode in the office with the nurse looking on. They ushered me into the cardiac intensive care unit.

Next they gave me some noninvasive tests, took some photographs to see what was blocked up, and then I had an angioplasty. After a few days, they told me they had done their job, and now it was my turn. They suggested a cardiac rehab program, which was three one-hour sessions a week of exercise and lectures.

Once you get down there and up the other side, then you can engage your heart and mind. But during that health crisis, everything else is unimportant. Later, I realized I had been ignorant about a lot. I had never given any credence to my ancestry, for one thing, and there were cardiovascular problems that we knew of at least through my grandfather's and my father's era. I had never given it a thought. Now I set out to change my living habits. I gave up smoking. But that wasn't as hard as leaving off the gravy from my meat—that is, when I get to have any meat. But nothing was as tough as lowering my stress level. It's not easy to turn the key off to the things that pull you and push at you every day of your life.

> "I am totally in God's hands, but I still have to work as though it all depends on me."

I see my life as having a purpose, no matter what I do. I am totally in God's hands, but I still have to work as though it all depends on me. There is this power that supports me, and the love of my wife and my children superimposed on that.

I have prayed always. But I changed the word "always" from one word to two words: "all ways." I try to live my whole life as a prayer.

In my line of work as a hospital chaplain, people will ask me, "What do you have to do to hear God speak to you?" I say that you have to fine-tune your mind and intellect to get what is being communicated to you. It comes in your thoughts, even in your dreams. And it works.

Chapter Eight

Travel

> When you come to a fork
> in the road, take it.
>
> —Yogi Berra

Recommendations from Experienced Travelers

Interview

RECOMMENDATIONS FROM EXPERIENCED TRAVELERS

If you have a stable heart condition, you can travel internationally with very few restrictions, maintains W. Robert Lange, M.D., a cardiologist and author of *The International Health Guide for Senior Citizen Travelers*. Air travel is considered safe for most people who can walk a block or climb a flight of stairs without becoming breathless. While there are individual differences, most people are encouraged to hear that within three or four months after a heart attack with no complications, they can travel with their doctor's blessing.

Travel is usually not recommended for men and women with uncontrollable high blood pressure, severe angina, congestive heart failure, or for those who have had a heart attack within four weeks of the trip.

"A natural reaction of men and women who have had a heart attack is an anxiety of traveling," says Dr. Erika Sivarajan Froelicher, an epidemiologist. "Overcoming the fear of traveling after a heart attack can be difficult." She recommends talking to experienced travelers with heart conditions.

Plan your trip more carefully than before. Make a list of every hotel and places you will be visiting. Many hotel dining rooms and restaurants in the United States are very familiar with specific diets. If you need specific services in your room, such as a refrigerator for medications, call the hotel as soon as possible. Don't rely on guidebooks or other information that may be outdated.

Outside of the U.S., travel can be more challenging, but many tour groups and hotel chains are familiar with the needs of travelers with disabilities and medical conditions. Thousands of travelers with heart conditions have been pleased with the tours of the American Association of Retired Persons and other groups.

Here are recommendations for planning a trip from men and women with heart conditions who are seasoned travelers.

• **Choose trips similar in pace to your schedule at home.** Plan trips in which you spend several nights in one place. If the climate is either hot, cold, or humid, arrange for heated or air-conditioned hotels and cars.

• **Go through the trip in your mind.** Try to identify the stresses and strains of the trip. To avoid feeling rushed, create a schedule with ample time for all of your activities.

• **Treat yourself to whatever services will make the trip more enjoyable.** Budget for tipping porters to help you with your luggage. At the airport, arrange for the services of a motorized cart that carries passengers between gates, or consider ordering a wheelchair to meet you at the gate to save walking long distances.

• **Travel with a companion who, like you, has a copy of your medical records.** Carry a copy of your electrocardiogram (ECG), a summary of your condition, a list of current medications and equipment, and your doctor's telephone number. Your doctor should be able to give you the names of several board-certified cardiologists in the cities you are visiting, as well as the names of the best medical facilities.

• **Check your insurance coverage before going on your trip.** Medicare and many insurance plans do not have coverage outside of the United States. Several companies and organizations provide temporary health insurance for travelers overseas. In addition, these companies provide trip cancellation insurance. Check with any local insurance agent or travel agent, or contact either Travel

Assistance International, 1133 15th Street NW, Suite 400, Washington, DC 20005; 800-821-2828; or Access America, Inc., P.O. Box 1188, Richmond, VA 23230; 800-284-8300.

• **Contact a travel agent who understands your travel needs.** The National Rehabilitation Information Center, 8455 Colesville Road, Suite 935, Silver Spring, MD 20910-3319; 800-346-2742 (Voice/TDD), has a list of experienced travel agents for travelers with disabilities, and related travel information.

• **Request an aisle seat.** On the plane you can get up every thirty minutes, walk about the cabin, and have easy access to the rest room if you are on the aisle. Raise and lower your legs to stimulate circulation. Stretch in your seat throughout the trip.

• **Arrange to have food prepared to your taste.** Forty-eight hours in advance of a plane trip, request a fruit plate or another low-salt, low-cholesterol, low-fat item from among a wide selection of heart-healthy foods available on most major airlines. Double-check to make sure they have your request. During the trip, drink lots of water and low-sodium tomato juice, and avoid carbonated beverages and alcohol.

• **Keep your medications with you in a carry-on bag.** Have everything you need for the next twenty-four hours, including supplies and medication in case your baggage becomes lost. Carry enough medication with you, plus a little extra. If your travel takes you overseas, make sure to have medications labeled with your name, especially if they are narcotics, tranquilizers, or sleeping pills. If you carry syringes, have a note from your doctor in case you are questioned by customs.

• **Keep the same medication schedule as you would at home.** If you change times zones, especially if it's for a short time, maintain the same schedule.

• **Balance activity with rest as you would at home.** In warm climates, use the early morning and late afternoon for walking and sight-seeing. Give yourself a day or two to adjust to the climate.

• **Sign up with Medic Alert's international registry.** Any doctor can call in and, by giving your membership number, get a list of your medications and your condition from anywhere in the world. For more about Medic Alert, see page 156.

• **Avoid metal security detectors if you have a pacemaker.** It is not unusual for someone with a pacemaker to ask to be checked by security rather than going through a metal security detector. Have enough battery life in the pacemakers pulse generator to last for your trip. Many pacemakers monitored by electronic telephone diagnostic systems do not transmit internationally. Make alternative arrangements for monitoring while traveling.

• **Would you be more comfortable during the flight with supplementary oxygen?** If so, airlines can provide oxygen for about $50, if you give them forty-eight-hours' notice. The airline will want written instructions from your doctor specifying if the oxygen delivery should be continuous or intermittent, as well as the prescribed flow rate. If you become short of breath at any time during a flight, you can ask the flight attendant for oxygen.

From an interview with a seventy-year-old man with a congestive heart condition

No matter your economic status, when you're sick and trying to recover, you need help from your family and friends, neighbors, professionals. Whoever has something to offer, you probably can use it.

You also need very deep pockets to pay for everything that isn't covered by insurance. Like the private ambulance that took me to the hospital. That cost $650. What are you going to do? If you need something badly enough, you find the money.

In my family, we all pool our money and pay the bills; not right away, but we pay up. When I went to see my doctor after I first came home, I needed a car service. It costs more than if I took my car, but after my heart attack, I wasn't allowed to drive for a while, and then I found it hard to get a parking space near my doctor's office. That tired me out so much, it gave me chest pains. I've learned to ask myself what causes my angina and try to work with it.

Money worries . . . that's always going to be there, even though my wife and I both work. The added costs when you get sick have to be budgeted. Some medicine and supplies are not fully covered, and I needed a physical therapist, and someone to help me when my wife went back to work. It all adds up.

"My family and I figure out how to get the most out of every dollar we spend. I want my money's worth no matter who or what it is."

My family and I figure out how to get the most out of every dollar we spend. I want my money's worth no matter who or what it is. I understand that professionals are selling their time and services. And what with me taking four different types of medication and the drugstores in my neighborhood varying as much as fifteen dollars in price on a single prescription, I go comparison shopping— sometimes even by phone—for my medicine.

I know what I'm entitled to, and the benefits from my HMO, and what's tax-deductible. My accountant helps a lot, and so does the woman who handles the benefits where I work. I call anyway to double-check. I'm keeping track of everything—what we paid, what's outstanding, etc.—and that helps me know what I'm up to. I think, on the whole, by carefully and thoroughly tracking our expenses, we're doing a pretty good job of stretching our medical dollar to the maximum.

Chapter Nine

Information, Services, and Products

Experience is not what happens to you; it is what you do with what happens to you.

—ALDOUS HUXLEY

Finding Community Resources

Home Care Services

Support for Caregiving Families

Support Groups

Psychological Counseling

Books for Heart and Mind

Audiotapes

Newsletters and other Publications

Interview

Finding Community Resources

When you need outside help but you aren't sure where to go for it or even what to ask for, a local organization that provides information and refers you to the appropriate organization is your best bet.

• **The telephone book is a good starting place.** Most phone books have a section of blue pages listing area agencies. In the yellow pages look under "Social and Human Services." Many communities and organizations also publish telephone directories that list only community support services. Looking at the listings of organizations usually helps to begin the networking process that is usually necessary to find what you want.

• **Local chapters of the American Heart Association have consumer information.** Organizations that serve people with a particular medical condition make referrals to community organizations, services, support groups, and visitors' programs, loan equipment, and provide counseling for individuals and families.

• **An Area Agency on Aging is an excellent resource for local organizations.** The Agency funds a variety of community services for the elderly. More about their services can be found on page 178.

• **Many home health care services are available in every state.** Public agencies, private organizations, and volunteer groups all provide services. There is no central agency that coordinates or evaluates all home care services.

The hospital discharge planner, your doctor, family, and friends can recommend home care agencies. If nursing and physical therapy have been ordered by your doctor, and you know the services will be approved by your insurance, you will need to use only those agencies approved by your insurance in order to be reimbursed.

• **Independent Living Centers are another fine resource.** Two hundred nonresidential centers run by disabled consumers coordinate or directly provide services such as transportation, a list of experienced personal care aides, information about accessibility, job counseling, psychological support services to families, and peer support. To find a nearby independent living center, call or write to Southern Tier Independence Center, 107 Chenango Street, Binghamton, NY 13901; (607) 724-2111.

• **Community Ys have low-cost cardiac exercise programs.** Classes, workshops, and programs for families at the Y are low-cost, and include water aerobics, nutrition, and weight-loss programs.

• **The Health Information Center, 800-336-4797, locates health information through the appropriate national organizations, associations, clearinghouses, and self-help support groups.** The Center is a program of the Office of Disease Prevention and Health Promotion, P.O. Box 1133, Washington, DC 20013.

• **Local Mental Health Associations are a referral resource.** The associations will make referrals to their member therapists. For more about mental health resources, see pages 183–84.

HOME CARE SERVICES

Nursing

If nursing services have been ordered by your doctor, or you and your family want a nurse, many options are available.

The private-duty Nursing Registry at the hospital will arrange for a nurse to accompany you home. Your local Nursing Bureau or Nursing Registry, whose address and phone number can be found in the yellow pages, will send a nurse to your home upon a simple phone request.

Visiting Nurse Associations and other nonprofit groups will usually send a nurse for a single, approximately one-hour visit, but the for-profit, private home care agencies will also arrange for shift work, if it is requested, just like in the hospital.

Shift work is usually in eight-hour blocks of time—7 A.M. to 3 P.M., 3 P.M. to 11 P.M., and 11 P.M. to 7 A.M. Especially during postoperative care, several home visits can give the family the confidence to manage. The nurses can evaluate and assess the care that is needed and teach any of the needed procedures. If the nursing services are reimbursable by insurance, the home care or nursing agency must be from an approved agency. For more about home care services, see pages 66 and 180–81.

Personal Care Aides

In any community, several sources exist for finding people who are willing to provide personal care assistance. By calling any full-service home care agency, you should be able to get a personal aide. The agencies interview and train the aide, and a nurse supervises from time to time in your home.

Most agencies will not send a personal care aide for less than four hours a day. If you want to interview the person beforehand, you may be charged for a minimum of four hours, so ask about this.

See page 66 for more about recruiting and training a personal care aide outside the auspices of an agency.

Physical Therapy

The American Physical Therapy Association, 1111 North Fairfax Street, Alexandria, VA 22314, (800) 999-2782 and (703) 684-2782. Registered physical therapists and assistants are licensed and regulated by the states. The Association is a good source of information about physical therapy and will refer you to your state association. Most states require that you be referred by a doctor. The department of physical therapy in hospitals and rehabilitation centers are good referral sources, as are members of coronary care clubs.

Nutritionists

Almost anyone can call himself or herself a nutritionist, since licensing is not required. Many sources offer sound nutritional information and advice.

Most legitimate nutritionists are likely to be members of the Society of Nutritional Education, the American Institute of Nutrition, or the American Association of Clinical Nutrition, which have strict entry requirements.

Registered dietitians have completed a prescribed

course of study in dietetics or nutrition, plus an internship in a hospital or other professional setting.

Increasingly, registered dietitians are setting up private practices as consulting dietitians and counsel clients who are self-referred or referred by doctors. You can find a listing in the yellow pages or with the nutrition clinic of a local hospital. Local chapters of the American Heart Association will refer you to a dietitian or nutritionist.

For the names of registered dietitians, contact the American Dietetic Association, 216 West Jackson Boulevard, Suite 800, Chicago, IL 60606. The consumer hot line is (800) 366-1655 or (312) 899-0040. Or send your request plus a stamped self-addressed business-size envelope to the Association.

Occupational Therapy

Occupational therapists help with daily living activities, and are particularly helpful in finding ways to conserve energy in everyday chores at home, as well as in the workplace. The American Occupational Therapy Association, Inc., P.O. Box 1725, Rockville, MD 20849-1725, (301) 948-9626, is a professional association that has information and printed materials about occupational therapy. Occupational therapists may require that you be referred by your doctor. The occupational therapy departments of hospitals and rehabilitation centers are a good source of referrals.

SUPPORT FOR CAREGIVING FAMILIES

It is estimated that as many as 10 million people between ages forty-five and sixty care for a dependent relative or older adult. Recent studies show that about 65 percent of all American caregivers are under sixty-five; over 40 percent hold full-time jobs.

Here are some information resources for families:

• **The hospital social work department offers information about community services.** While you are in the hospital you can get a wealth of free information from the social work department. The hospital discharge planner, with your permission, will arrange for home care services.

• **Local libraries have useful resources.** You are likely to find the names, addresses, and telephone numbers of community organizations, as well as a listing of the services available in your area.

• **Your doctor, his or her nurse, or assistants may recommend organizations and services.** You may get good leads on services that others have used and told the staff about.

• **The Area Agency on Aging (AAA) sets up needed nonmedical services.** The AAA is a governmental agency that funds community home-delivered meals, free transportation to doctors' offices, shopping and housekeeping help, and social activities, among other functions. They can refer families to companies that manage and provide professional home care services, including nurses, personal care aides, and physiotherapists. Some AAA offices provide financial-planning assistance, or will advise you where to find it. You can find the agency listed in the yellow pages of the phone directory under "Social Service Organizations" or "Guide to Human Services."

• **The National Rehabilitation Information Center (NARIC) is a library and information center on dis-**

ability and rehabilitation information. NARIC collects and disseminates information from books, journal articles, and audiovisuals on all aspects of rehabilitation and disability, including independent living, employment, medical rehabilitation, and legislation.

ABLEDATA, a national database of products and rehabilitation equipment from domestic and international sources, is available by calling NARIC 800-346-2741, or writing NARIC, 8455 Colesville Road, Suite 935, Silver Spring, MD 20910-3319.

• **Senior centers provide programs and respite care for primary caregivers.** Especially for family members who need to work outside the home, senior centers have programs of classes, lectures, and outings. These usually are free, except for a charge for meals. A particular center may be for chronically ill elders who need a place to go for minimal medical care and supervised therapy, as well as socializing.

• **Church and synagogue bulletin boards and newsletters list the support organizations and programs available to families.** Houses of worship offer spiritual support as well as community programs.

• **Telephone reassurance and friendly visiting are reassuring and often essential for someone living alone.** Many churches, synagogues, hospital auxiliaries, and volunteer organizations have established telephone projects. Visiting services are offered by a variety of volunteer agencies and organizations, including some labor unions who offer them as benefits for their retired members.

• **Transportation services, especially for elderly citizens, are available in many communities.** Car, bus, and van services, some equipped for disabled passengers and

wheelchair users, are provided by various community organizations. Taxi services may offer discounts for senior
citizens.

• **Family Service America (FSA) provides family counseling services.** Through its two hundred member agencies nationwide, this organization provides families with
information and referral services, as well as counseling
and support groups. Write to FSA at 11700 West Lake Park
Drive, Milwaukee, WI 53224. Call 800-221-2681 for the
location of the agency serving your community.

• **Adult Day Care centers provide care for older people
who can no longer remain at home alone but who do
not need skilled nursing care.** This is a fairly new concept, and centers are not available in all communities.
Some facilities are not-for-profit, and get federal and community assistance. Others are privately owned and oper-
ated for profit.

• **Private geriatric-care managers assist a family member who lives at a distance or who works at a full-time
job.** Care managers are social workers, nurses, or psychologists who have private practices to counsel and assist families in planning for long-term care. They arrange
for home health care as needed, such as visiting nurses;
occupational, physical, speech, or other therapists; and
personal care and homemaker workers.

The two following national organizations can provide
help in locating social workers: Aging Network Services,
Inc., 4400 East-West Hwy, Suite 907, Bethesda, MD
20814, (301) 657-4329, has a national network of 250 geri-
atric social workers; and the National Association of Professional Geriatric-Care Managers, 655 N. Alvernon Way,
Suite 108, Tucson, AZ 85711, (602) 881-8008, sets

standards for the profession and acts as a national referral service.

• **Children of Aging Parents,** Woodburne Office Campus, Suite 302A, Levittown, PA 19057, (215) 945-6900. This is a national clearinghouse for caregiving families.

• **Elder Support Network provides a variety of services based on ability to pay.** With 146 affiliate organizations, this service of the Association of Jewish Family and Children's Agencies offers Meals-on-Wheels, respite care, telephone assurance, friendly visiting, home care, and transportation.

Another organization, Eldercare Locators, helps callers obtain information toll-free about community services available throughout the country. Call 800-677-1116.

• **Hospice care is provided in homes.** For information about hospice programs, contact the National Hospice Organization, 1901 North Moore Street, Suite 901, Arlington, VA 22209, (703) 243-5900.

• **Well Spouse Foundation is the support group for well caregiving spouses.** One hundred support groups meet to exchange information and support one another. Meetings have invited speakers, discussions, personal exchanges, with the focus on the well spouse. The $15 membership fee includes a newsletter. Call or write Well Spouse Foundation, P.O. Box 801, New York, NY 10023, (212) 724-7209.

• **American Association of Retired Persons**, 601 E Street NW; Washington, DC 20049; (202) 434-2277. The world's largest nonprofit, nonpartisan organization enhancing the quality of life for older people. The organization offers discounts, free publications, a mail-order pharmacy service, and travel service, to name a few of their services. The $8-a-year membership includes the *AARP News Bulletin* and *Modern Maturity*.

• **The People's Medical Society is an organization working to protect medical rights.** For a description of their services, address, and telephone number, see page 37.

SUPPORT GROUPS

• **The American Self-Help Clearinghouse,** St. Clare's-Riverside Medical Center, Denville, NJ 07834, (201) 625-7101; TDD 625-9053. Callers on the center's helpline are given information about specific groups of interest to them.

• **Mended Hearts,** 7320 Greenville Avenue, Dallas, TX 75231-4596, (214) 706-7272, is an organization with 225 chapters for men and women with heart conditions, and their families. Meetings feature invited speakers who talk on a variety of health issues, with interactive discussions, rap sessions, and social get-togethers. Individual dues: $15; family membership: $22; membership includes their newsletter, *Heartbeat*.

• **Coronary Club, Inc.,** 9500 Euclid Avenue, Cleveland, OH 44195, (216) 444-3690, with five affiliates, meets to educate and to give mutual support to people with heart conditions and their families. The organization offers a monthly newsletter, *Heartline*, covering a wide range of subjects. A subscription is $29.

In addition, many organizations and hospitals sponsor coronary care clubs and support groups. The American Heart Association can direct you to groups in your community.

• **The American Chronic Pain Association**, P.O. Box 850, Rocklin, CA 95677, (916) 632-0922, is a self-help organization with over 500 groups internationally, with information and other services for people who have chronic pain, and their families.

• An estimated fifteen million people attend weekly twelve-step support programs. Another one hundred million people—friends and family—encourage them. **Alcoholics Anonymous, Smokers Anonymous, Overeaters Anonymous, Narcotics Anonymous, and Alanon** (for a caregiving family member or friend) are listed in the telephone book.

PSYCHOLOGICAL COUNSELING

Your doctor, dentist, and other health care professionals are good resources for therapists.

Local Mental Health Association offices make referrals of practitioners and support groups in the area.

Your state psychology licensing board, which may be listed in your telephone book under state government, is another source of referral.

Hospitals, medical centers, and the rehabilitation institutions affiliated with academic medical schools are referral resources. Most hospitals have therapists on their staff who provide individual and family therapy, as well as stress-reduction programs, biofeedback, relaxation techniques, support, and peer counseling.

• **American Association of Sex Educators, Counselors and Therapists,** 435 N. Michigan Avenue, Suite 1717, Chicago, IL 60611, (312) 644-0828, offers referrals to sex counselors experienced in sexuality problems resulting from physical illness.

Local chapters of the American Psychiatric Association make referrals.

Medical social services are provided by social workers who act as information and referral sources, but in addition to finding the resources, can also provide general counseling and emotional support. Most home health care agencies and Visiting Nurse Associations have social workers on staff to help identify your particular needs.

Books for Heart and Mind

Of the countless books available on heart conditions, these are but a few of the many that are outstanding.

Food

COOLEY, DENTON, AND CAROLYN MOORE
Eat Smart for a Healthy Heart Cookbook
Barron's, 1992
   A distinguished heart surgeon and a dietitian bring together menus and recipes that please the most demanding

gourmet yet conform to the requirements of people with heart conditions.

DEBAKEY, MICHAEL E., ANTONIO M. GROTTO, JR., LYNN W. SCOTT, AND JOHN P. FOREYT
The Living Heart: Brand Name Shopper's Guide
Master Media, 1992
> Take Dr. DeBakey's book on your next shopping trip. A guide to thousands of brand-name products low in fat that have the blessings of a renowned cardiac surgeon.

ESHELMAN, RUTH (EDITOR)
The American Heart Association Cookbook
4th Edition, Ballantine, 1988
> Best recipes submitted by thousands of friends, volunteers, and nutritionists of the American Heart Association chapters and affiliates.

KUSHI, MICHIO, WITH ALEX JACK
Diet for a Strong Heart
St. Martin's Press, 1985
> Macrobiotic dietary guidelines for prevention and healing of high blood pressure, heart attack, and stroke.

PISCATELLA, JOSEPH
Controlling Your Fat Tooth
Workman, 1991
> The author of *Don't Eat Your Heart Out Cookbook* and *Choices for a Healthy Heart* creates a simple, do-it-yourself approach to managing fat in your diet without feeling deprived.

PRITIKIN, ROBERT
The New Pritikin Program
Pocket Books, 1991
> The Pritikin eating plan and pioneering life-style approach to controlling, and reversing, most heart conditions. See

the list of newsletters on page 194 for more information about Pritikin programs.

SCHWARTZ, GEORGE R., AND MARTHA ROSE SHULMAN
Healthy Company Menus with Great Style
Bantam Books, 1991
  Martha Shulman creates delicious, light, and less rich recipes.

SPEAR, RUTH
Low Fat and Loving It
Bantam Books, 1991
  How to lower your fat intake and still eat the foods you love.

Heart Conditions: Cause and Cure

COHAN, CAROL, JUNE B. PIMM, AND JAMES R. JUDE
A Patient's Guide to Heart Surgery: Understanding the Practical and Emotional Aspects of Heart Surgery
Harper Perennial, 1991
  Beyond the basics of what most people are told before undergoing heart surgery.

GOLDMAN, MARTIN
The Handbook of Heart Drugs: A Consumer's Guide to Safe and Effective Use
Henry Holt, 1992
  A cardiologist explains more than ninety of the most common heart drugs in an understandable way, along with what you should expect from your doctor and yourself.

GORDON, NEIL F., AND LARRY W. GIBBONS
The Cooper Cardiac Rehabilitation Program
Simon & Schuster, 1992
  A cardiac rehabilitation survival guide that explains what has taken place and how to take care of yourself.

FRIEDMAN, MEYER, AND DIANE ULMER
Treating Type A Behavior and Your Heart
Fawcett, 1985
> Describes the program designed to help men who have had
> a heart attack reduce their Type A behavior.

HUBBARD, STEVE G., AND GARY FERGUSON
Recovering from Coronary Bypass Surgery
Harper Paperbacks, 1992
> A revealing and reassuring handbook to bypass surgery
> and recovery.

LEGATO, MARIANNE J., AND CAROL COLEMAN
*The Female Heart: The Truth About Women and Coronary Artery
Disease*
Simon & Schuster, 1991
> Replaces with vital information the myth that heart dis-
> ease is only a man's problem.

ORNISH, DEAN
Dr. Dean Ornish's Program for Reversing Heart Disease
Ballantine, 1992
> Covers managing stress through meditation, psychologi-
> cal counseling, peer support, with guidelines for exercise
> and diet. Excellent low-fat, heart-healthy meals. See the
> list of audiotapes on page 193 for more about Dr. Ornish's
> program.

SOTILE, WAYNE M.
*Intimacy and Heart Illness: How Caring Relationships
Aid Recovery*
Johns Hopkins, 1992
> A reassuring consumer's guide to common concerns about
> sex, intimacy, and heart illness. See the list of audiotapes
> on page 192 for more about Dr. Sotile's program.

WILLIAMS, REDFORD
The Trusting Heart: Great News About Type A Behavior
Times Books/Random House, 1989
  A detailed review of the research showing that hostility is
  the only unhealthy component of Type A behavior.

WILLIAMS, REDFORD, AND VIRGINIA WILLIAMS
*Anger Kills: Seventeen Strategies for Reducing the Hostility That
Can Harm Your Health*
Times Books/Random House, 1992
  How to tell if you have a hostile personality, its effect on
  your heart, and what to do about it if you do.

ZARET, BARRY L., MARVIN MOSER, AND LAWRENCE S. COHEN
Yale University School of Medicine, Heart Book
Hearst Books, 1992
  The most comprehensive and well-illustrated guide to the
  symptoms, diagnoses, tests, and treatments of all heart
  conditions.

Eliminating Physical and Emotional Risk Factors

Available from local chapters of the American Cancer
Society:
I Quit Kit. A Self-Help Smoking Program

These pamphlets are available from local chapters of the
American Lung Association:
A Lifetime of Freedom from Smoking.
Freedom from Smoking in 20 Days.
Help a Friend to Stop Smoking.

BURNS, DAVID D.
The Feeling Good Handbook: Using the New Mood Therapy in Everyday Life
NAL-Dutton, 1990
> The author of *Feeling Good*, a best-seller on depression, now shows you how to develop self-esteem, enjoy greater intimacy, and overcome anxiety, fears, and phobias.

FASSEL, DIANE
Working Ourselves to Death
Harper, 1992
> Looks at the problems of workaholism and the strategies to overcome it.

FERGUSON, TOM, M.D.
The No-Nag, No-Guilt, Do-It-Your-Own-Way Guide to Quitting Smoking
Ballantine Books, 1987
> The steps to take in becoming a permanent nonsmoker, and information for families and friends who want to support the effort. See the list of audiotapes on quitting smoking.

LERNER, HARRIET GOLDHOR
The Dance of Anger: A Women's Guide to Changing the Patterns of Intimate Relationships
HarperCollins, 1985
> From a respected authority on the psychology of women and the change in families, an enlightening study on women and anger.

LIEBELT, ROBERT
Straight Talk About Alcoholism
Pharos Books, 1992
> A doctor explains the causes of alcoholism, its effects, and what you can do about it.

MOHS-CATALANO, ELLEN M.
Chronic Pain Control Work Book
New Harbinger, 1987
   Looks at understanding various types of pain and discusses home strategies to reduce pain and to cope with discomfort.

SELIGMAN, MARTIN, E.P.
Learned Optimism
Pocket Books, 1990
   A guide that outlines easy-to-follow techniques that have helped thousands of people rise above pessimism and the depression that accompanies negative thoughts.

SHEALY, C. NORMAN
The Pain Game
Celestial Arts, 1976
   The physical reasons for pain are explained, as well as its mental effect on people. The author reveals the games doctors and patients play, and shows how to control pain.

TAVRIS, CAROL
Anger: The Misunderstood Emotion
Simon & Schuster, 1989
   This widely read book dispels many of the myths about anger.

TUBESING, DONALD A.
Kicking Your Stress Habits
Whole Person Associates, Inc., 1981
P.O. Box 3151, Duluth, MN 55803; (218) 727-0500
   A workbook that helps you identify your beliefs, values, and goals, to focus on what really matters, and in so doing, to worry less about irrelevant events or concerns.

Mind–Body Medicine

BENSON, HERBERT
The Relaxation Response
William Morrow, 1975
> The leading self-help guide to the easy-to-learn quieting state.

BENSON, HERBERT, ELLEN M. STUART, AND THE STAFF OF THE MIND/BODY MEDICAL INSTITUTE
The Wellness Book: The Comprehensive Guide to Maintaining Health and Treating Stress-Related Illness
Birch Lane Press, 1992
> A workbook following the program of the Mind/Body Medical Institute, it includes stress management, exercise, and nutrition—to provide a complete guide for enhancing health and dealing with cardiovascular and most other illnesses. For audiotapes of the program, see page 193.

BORYSENKO, JOAN
Minding the Body, Mending the Mind
Addison-Wesley, 1987
> Draws upon professional and personal experiences in mind–body research. See the list of audiotapes for more about the author's healing approach that embraces the mind, body, and spirit.

COUSINS, NORMAN
The Healing Heart
Avon, 1983
> A heart attack survivor tells you how to overcome panic, release your body's miraculous healing powers, and rediscover living.

KABAT-ZINN, JON
*Full Catastrophe Living: Using the Wisdom of Your Body and
Mind to Face Stress, Pain and Illness*
Delacorte Press, 1990
> A detailed, step-by-step manual of mindfulness meditation
> and its applications for mainstream Americans. For a list
> of accompanying meditation audiotapes led by Dr. Kabat-
> Zinn, see page 193. Also by Dr. Kabat-Zinn: *Wherever You
> Go, There You Are: Mindfulness Meditation in Everyday Life,
> Meditations for Daily Living*. Discusses ways to integrate
> mindfulness into one's daily life.

AUDIOTAPES

Cardiac Couples,
> c/o Wayne M. Sotile, Ph.D., 1396 Old Mill Circle, Winston-
> Salem, NC 27103; (919) 765-3032. Audiotapes include: Sex-
> ual Aspects of Cardiac Rehabilitation; The Couple's Jour-
> ney: The Challenge of Change in Marriage; Men in
> Recovery: Sex, Intimacy and Health; Thriving, Not Just
> Surviving: Cardiac Rehabilitation Is More Than Just Exer-
> cise.

Self-Care Productions,
> c/o Great Performance, 14964 NW Greenbrier Pkwy., Bea-
> verton, OR 97006-5797; 800-433-3803. Audiotapes include
> "Helping Smokers Get Ready to Quit" by Dr. Tom Fer-
> guson, which follows the guilt-free, self-care approach to
> quitting smoking. Dr. Ferguson's book, *The No-Nag, No-
> Guilt, Do-It-Your-Own-Way Guide to Quitting Smoking*, is
> also available directly from Great Performance.

The Mind/Body Medical Institute, Division of Behavioral Medicine, New England Deaconess Hospital,
185 Pilgrim Road, Boston, MA 02215; (617) 632-9530. Audiotapes used in their program for people dealing with cardiac rehabilitation, hypertension, pain, and other stress-related medical conditions.

Mind/Body Health Sciences, Inc.,
393 Dixon Road, Salina Route, Boulder, CO 80302; (303) 440-8460. Tapes designed to promote inner wisdom and healing. A quarterly newsletter gives information about workshops, and trainings by Joan and Myrin Borysenko.

Stress Reduction Tapes,
P.O. Box 547, Lexington, MA 02173. Mindfulness meditation practice tapes led by Jon Kabet-Zinn and used at the University of Massachusetts Medical Center's Stress Reduction Clinic.

Dr. Dean Ornish's Program for Reversing Heart Disease,
Audiotapes and information from Dr. Dean Ornish's program which combines a mind–body approach, life-style modifications, and supportive professional counseling and peer support are available in bookstores.

Peaceful Warrior Services,
P.O. Box 6148—Dept. NOM, San Rafael, CA 94903; (415) 491-0301. "When the Going Gets Tough," "Rules for Being Human," and "The Peaceful Warrior" are among the many tapes offered to expand awareness, inspire action, and uplift the spirit.

NEWSLETTERS AND OTHER PUBLICATIONS

Tufts University Diet & Nutrition Letter (monthly) from Tufts, P.O. Box 5787, Boulder, CO 80322-7857; (800) 274-7581.

Harvard Heart Letter (monthly) from Harvard Heart Letter, P.O. Box 420234, Palm Coast, FL 32142-0234.

University of California Berkeley Wellness Letter (monthly) from University of California, Berkeley Wellness Letter, P.O. Box 359148, Palm Coast, FL 32035.

Pritikin Vantage Point (monthly) from Pritikin Systems, Inc., 1910 Ocean Front Walk, Santa Monica, CA 90405. To learn about the Pritikin Longevity Centers and their program, call 800-421-9911.

Food News for Consumers (4 issues per year)—published by the USDA Food Safety and Inspection Service. Order from Superintendent of Documents, U.S. Government Printing Office, Washington, D.C. 20402. For a listing of "Publications for Sale," contact Human Nutrition Information Service, USDA, 6505 Belcrest Road, Hyattsville, MD 20782; (301) 436-8498.

From an interview with a forty-nine-year-old man who had a heart transplant

When you are in the hospital, people give you flowers—glorious, wonderful bouquets. You get cards to hang up. You get visits and all kinds of nice things, and that's good because you need that.

But when you leave the hospital, you need something else. And chances are that most of the flowers will be thrown out, the candy will be given to the nurses, and most of the cards will be filed away in order to write thank-you notes. What you need then is more flowers, more visits, more positive attention and affirmation. You also need conversation, and discussions aimed toward the future you have earned. You need to know that you are thought of in terms of having a future, and your life is your rightful reward for having left the hospital.

"There's no telling who or what it will be that gives you the will and determination to go forward—it's your openness to its reception that counts."

How you go through that tunnel of transition and come out the other end, how you feel about what has happened to you, and who urges you on, makes all the difference. It could be your wife or husband, children, grandchildren, friends of many years, God, or people you meet with similar experiences to yours. There's no telling who or what it will be that gives you the will and determination to go forward—it's your openness to its reception that counts.

Afterword

If you have been using this book, you have made the transition from the hospital to your home. You have steadily regained your strength and recuperated in various ways.

You've done this with the help of your family, and learned when and how to call on them for help. You've taken charge of your health with the guidance of your doctors and other professionals.

You've learned to set goals, monitor your diet and exercise, stop smoking, become aware of the cause of daily stress, and to use relaxation techniques. You've become adept at filling in charts and making lists. Chances are, too, that you've developed a few strategies of your own.

All of the life-style modifications that are recommended for you are actually no different from what doctors prescribe for people who want to *prevent* heart disease. In fact, the healthy choices that you are making can influence family members, friends, and coworkers to take a good, hard look at their own health habits, diets, and exercise regimes. If this book has helped you to improve the quality of your own life and the lives of others, it will have served its purpose well.

About the Authors

Florence Weiner has written several books about survival and disability, including *No Apologies: A Guide to Living with a Disability, Help for the Handicapped Child,* and *How to Survive in New York with Children.* She is a disability rights activist and cofounder with Harriet Bell of the Polio Information Center.

Mathew H. M. Lee, M.D., F.A.C.P., has been a rehabilitation physician for thirty-five years and is currently Medical Director at the Rusk Institute of Rehabilitation Medicine, New York University Medical Center, in New York City. He is also Professor, Clinical Rehabilitation Medicine, and Clinical Professor, Behavioral Sciences and Community Health, at New York University. Dr. Lee is the editor of *Rehabilitation, Music and Human Well-Being.*

Harriet Bell, Ph.D., was formerly a member of the New York State Board of Nursing, past president of the Auxiliary and the Community Board at Goldwater Memorial Hospital, Roosevelt Island, New York, where she lived for twenty-five years after contracting polio. Dr. Bell now lives in the community.

Numbers to Call in an Emergency

**(in LARGE, BOLD print, write the name and
the number of the people
you need to call in an emergency)**

NAME (Your Doctor):

TELEPHONE NO.:

NAME (Emergency Medical Service):

TELEPHONE NO.:

NAME (Hospital):

TELEPHONE NO.:

NAME (Family Member at Work):

TELEPHONE NO.:

NAME:

TELEPHONE NO.:

NAME:

TELEPHONE NO.:

NAME:

TELEPHONE NO.:

Notes

Notes

Index

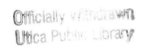